Breast Health Exposed

21 Secrets Most Doctors Will Never Tell You About Your Breasts

Jan Janzen

Women Empowering Women Inc.
Vancouver, British Columbia, Canada

Breast Health Exposed: 21 Secrets Most Doctors
Will Never Tell You About Your Breasts

Copyright © 2010 Jan Janzen. All rights reserved.

No part of this publication may be reproduced or transmitted in any form or by any means electronic or mechanical, including photocopying, recording, or by any information storage and retrieval system, without written permission from the copyright owner.

Printed in the United States

Printed on Recycled Paper

Cover Design by Kickstart Communications
Illustrations by Chris Price
Formatting by Diane Mendez

Library and Archives Canada Cataloguing in Publication
    Janzen, Jan, 1961-
    Breast health exposed : 21 secrets most doctors will never tell you
    about your breasts / Jan Janzen.
    Includes bibliographical references.
    ISBN 978-0-9810754-2-6
    1. Breast–Care and hygiene. 2. Breast–Diseases–Prevention.
    3. Women–Health and hygiene. I. Title.
    RG491.J35 2010 618.1'9 C2010-905514-4

Publisher: Women Empowering Women Inc.

For information contact Women Empowering Women Inc. at info@womenempoweringwomen.biz

For a complete list of all the resources used for this book, please visit www.breasthealthrevolution.com/resources/BreastHealthExposed

Dedication

This book is dedicated to all of the breast health ambassadors, who are championing a different way to breast health and is a celebration of the millions more who will join them.

There is a better way.

About the Author....

Jan Janzen

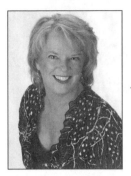

I bought my first franchise at the age of 19 and have been an entrepreneur for more than 29 years. My first book, *Devil with a Briefcase, 101 Success Secrets for the Spiritual Entrepreneur,* along with my Spiritual Entrepreneur CD series, have helped guide entrepreneurs who want it all—fun, values and profit in their businesses while making a difference in the world.

Getting off the Merry-Go-Round, How to Create the Life You Want Without the Fear, Doubt and Guilt chronicles my journey from almost bankrupt, homeless and divorced, to leading the most amazing life I live today. By healing the emotional issues that had plagued me from childhood, I have been able to forgive, move forward and create what I want in life.

I am also the best-selling author of a beautiful compilation of inspiring stories from 37 authors alongside myself. *Overcomers Inc. - True Stories of Hope, Courage and Inspiration* is the book every person needs on their bedside table.

My fifth book, *The Booby Trap: How Complacency is Costing Women Their Lives* is due out early 2011.

I'm a philanthropist and an activist, constantly looking for ways to improve the lives of women around the globe. *Breast Health Exposed – 21 Secrets Most Doctors Will Never Tell You About Your Breasts* is a contribution to a movement that involves education and empowerment.

I am blessed to spend most of the year in sunny places around the world, including Mexico, Sedona, Arizona and Guatemala, where I get to live a truly magical life that is abundant in love, joy, peace and prosperity, the very foundation of my work.

For more information visit www.janjanzen.com

For more information on The Breast Health Revolution visit
www.breasthealthrevolution.com

Table of Contents

Acknowledgments vii

Foreword by Brenda Eastwood ix

The Journey Begins 1

Secret #1: Avoid Root Canals 5

Secret #2: Wear Your Bra As Little As Possible 9

Secret #3: Get Your Lymphatic System Moving 13

Secret #4: Sweat it Out 17

Secret #5: Get Out in the Sunshine 21

Secret #6: Sleep in the Dark 25

Secret #7: Find Ways to Deal with Stress 29

Secret #8: Wash All New Clothes Before You Wear Them 33

Secret #9: Take Breast Health Back Into Your Own Hands 37

Secret #10: Get Alkaline 41

Secret #11: Watch What You Put On Your Body 45

Secret #12: Love Your Breasts 49

Secret #13: Mammography Can Cause Cancer 53

Secret #14: Choose Thermography 57

Secret #15: Check Your Iodine Level 61

Secret #16: Soy Is Not Good For Your Breasts 65

Secret #17: Get Rid of the Candida 69

Secret #18: Men Can Get Breast Cancer Too! 73

Secret #19: Your Weight is Putting Your Breasts at Risk 77

Secret #20: Antibiotics Can Lead to Cancer 81

Secret #21: The Scoop on Poop 85

A Salute to Healthy Breasts 89

Acknowledgements

Putting together a book is a massive project. Writing the book is only a very small part. Without an amazing team around any author, there would be no books!

A huge thanks to my amazing editor and formatter, Diane Mendez, who makes my books beautiful and easy to read. After reading hundreds of books over the last couple of years, I so appreciate Diane's unique formatting that continues to delight my readers.

Chris Price is such a delight to work with as he creates fabulous illustrations that make my books pleasurable to read. I also so appreciate that he never complains when I send illustrations back for revisions. Chris has a wonderful graciousness and energy about him that makes working with him an absolute breeze

Catherine Levan of Kickstart Communications has the patience of Job and then some. She patiently worked with me as she created the cover and was honest, diplomatic and always helpful as she guided and directed me constantly. A huge thank you!

Erin Stinson, my Virtual Assistant and Social Media Expert deserves huge kudos for keeping up with the fast pace, staying on top of things and making sure that everything in my business, including the marketing of this book runs smoothly. Not many could handle the demands but Erin does it with an expertise to be admired.

Rebekkah White, my webmaster and technology guru has built the websites to support this project. Working long hours to get it done on time, handling the challenging problems, patiently teaching me what only I can do and doing it all with a smile is Rebekkah's claim to fame. She is a god-send!

The newest member of my team, Kenda Morrison, who is looking after Public Relations, the Breast Health Exposed radio show and getting me ready for the media journey, deserves huge applause for jumping in midstream and swimming like crazy to catch up. I look forward to a long and fabulous relationship with this amazing woman!

This book would not have happened without the motivation and support of Alfred Pettersen and Tarl Robinson. As they hold the vision of a world without breast cancer for women, I appreciate their willingness to educate women about breast health. They could take the easy road and join the masses. Instead they are leading the path to a different way to breast health. I am in complete gratitude.

I have an amazing sister, who supports me by being there in so many practical ways so I can live the life I do. She is my only family member who loves me unconditionally, appreciates me for who I am and doesn't try to change me. That's a miracle! Julie, you have no idea how much it means to me. Thank you.

There have been countless times while researching breast cancer and breast health that I have thanked my mom. Although she passed away five years ago, I believe that her experience with breast cancer was so I could have the story, the passion and the determination that nobody would go through the fear she experienced after her diagnosis. Thank you, mom, for your constant support from above. I've felt it so many times.

To my dear, dear friend Brenda Eastwood who has supported this book in countless ways. She has seen my vision, fueled my passion and loved me through the ups and downs. Without her friendship and support, my life would be a whole lot less amazing! I love you lots!

To another dear friend, Monique McDonald, who told me to write this book when I didn't particularly want to. She never ceases to amaze me with her wisdom, her insight and her ability to see beyond the present. Thank you so much for believing wholeheartedly that there is a different way for women in the world and always making sure that I didn't shrink back from doing my part to make it happen. You are a rock in my life!

And to my special life partner, Greg, who has seen me through the tiredness, the stress, the long days and short nights. Who never stops believing in me and loving me for who I am and pushes me to greater successes. Thank you, my love, for being in my life, for being the amazing doctor you are, for doing your part to create breast health for every woman and smiling through it all. I love you!

And to all of the wonderful clients over the past six years who have given me the insight into the wonders, both physically and emotionally, of breast health. Thank you for trusting me to see what you needed so you could have an amazing life.

Foreword

Over the last 30 years, as a woman's health specialist, I have noticed that maintaining vibrant health has definitely become more challenging. When I started in private practice, I knew a lot less than I do now about health and nutrition, yet problems were much simpler to resolve.

Today, with stress in women's lives at an all-time high, an increasing amount of environmental toxins that have become impossible to avoid and the quality of our food sources seriously deteriorating, achieving optimal health has become very complex.

In my health coaching program today, I find that many women are confused about what to do to maintain healthy breasts. For most women, the fear of breast cancer is always looming in the background. And the women who are diagnosed with breast cancer are scared and overwhelmed.

That's why I love Jan's latest book, *Breast Health Exposed*. She has used her amazing talent for absorbing massive amounts of information, digesting it and then writing about it in a way the rest of the world can enjoy and comprehend. She has made keeping your breasts "happy and healthy" as she says, less intimidating than most books on breast health. She's made it simple. That doesn't mean it's always easy, because optimum health does take effort.

Breast health, like every other area of your body is not a one-size-fits-all program. That's why I also appreciate that Jan has given you 21 widely varying areas to investigate and implement in your life.

The beauty of working towards breast health is that you will also be rewarded with better health in other areas of your life. For example, I have seen Candida destroy a woman's health, and even cause death. So by understanding how Candida can put your breast health at risk, and eliminating this fungus from your body, not only will your breasts benefit, but your moods, energy, weight issues, sleep patterns and vaginal infections will improve as well. Those are great bonuses for taking care of your breasts.

So how reliable is this information? I find it lines up perfectly with everything that I have learned about breast health, and I can guarantee that given the controversial nature of the topic "what is best for your breasts" that Jan has thoroughly researched this book. This means you can trust the information and feel confident that you are doing the right thing by implementing any of her suggestions.

This is not a 'do as I say and not as I do' book. Jan practices what she preaches and it shows. If you were to follow her around for a few days, you would be extremely impressed with her healthy lifestyle choices. If you could keep up with her, you would see her vibrant glow and exuberant energy. Jan is truly a picture of GREAT health.

Jan wants all women to have what she has, healthy breasts and fabulous health. She has a clear vision that the tide on breast cancer statistics can be turned through knowledge, empowerment and action.

I believe Jan will accomplish her goal because she also brings to the table decades of experience as an accomplished businesswoman, a philanthropist and an activist with a passion for helping women. In all the years that I have known Jan, I've never seen her so committed or motivated by a mission like this one. She is driven beyond what I thought possible!

You know as well as I do that it isn't always who knows the most or who has the longest list of credentials, it is drive and passion that can affect the greatest change. We've seen this constantly throughout history and it certainly is the case today. Everyday ordinary people are doing extra-ordinary things that are making a difference in the world and changing history. I see that this book, *Breast Health Exposed*, can dramatically affect women's views on breast health and empower them to take breast health back into their own hands.

That knowledge and empowerment is long overdue. As I have seen women get sicker, more stressed and completely overwhelmed by their health issues, it's obvious that what we've been doing isn't working. You can't rely on your doctors to make you healthy. That is not their area of expertise. Unless your medical doctor has pursued a career in alternative medicine he/she has not trained in nutrition or any kind of preventative health care. What they know exceptionally well is disease management through prescription drugs and/or surgery.

Ignorance is NOT bliss. When you see the power you have to affect your own breast health, you will realize that the new focus and goal of every woman has to be on disease PREVENTION, not disease management.

Despite my vast knowledge in health and nutrition, I learned many things reading Jan's book so I am certain you will get much value from it. Please read it from cover to cover and then take action. These 21 secrets will not only change your breast health, they will change your life.

Yours in Total Health,

Brenda Eastwood

Women's Health Specialist
Registered Nutritional Consulting Practitioner
www.brendaeastwood.com

The Journey Begins

I was 31 years old when the words "breast cancer" first struck a chord of terror in me. I was sitting in the oncologist's office with my 70-year-old mother, who had just learned her biopsy was positive. As the doctor calmly informed her of the mastectomy date he had booked for her, he next turned to me and said, "And now young lady, you're at high risk." A mixture of anger and fear hurried us both out of his office.

My mother cancelled the surgery the day before she was due to have her breast removed and chose an unconventional course of treatment. Really quite amazing, considering she did it without the knowledge and resources the Internet would have afforded her today. Mom passed away in 2005 of natural causes, her breast cancer a forgotten issue.

For me however, it has been a different story. Just six years after hearing those ominous words in the oncologist's office, my husband found a lump in my right breast. I was terrified. I had recently watched a 32-year-old friend die of breast cancer. The following morning, I raced to the doctor who confirmed the lump. I then had the prescribed mammogram and a follow-up ultrasound, which indicated the lump was benign.

I breathed a sigh of relief and wondered if this was an indicator of negative things to come. Thankfully, over the last 12 years, I've learned a thing or two about breast health.

In 2008, while president of Plexus Worldwide, a network marketing company dedicated to breast health, I saw firsthand the pain and anguish of women diagnosed with breast cancer. I felt the passion of men and women on a mission to educate, inform and empower women to take breast health back into their own hands. It was a life-changing time for me, which has resulted, in part, in the writing of this book.

Breast Health Exposed is the first of a series of books on breast health. It is the foundation that every woman (and man) needs to understand about how we can eradicate breast cancer. It really is so unnecessary that every day, every 12 minutes, a woman dies of breast cancer. Lack of education, fear and greed are creating a travesty that future generations will surely look upon in horror.

As you read this book, you may be shocked or even skeptical as to whether these facts could really be true. Surely, if what I am telling you is the truth, your doctor, oncologist, a major cancer charity or the media would have advised you long before now. It may be easy to dismiss these 21 secrets as either completely outrageous or too easy to believe they can actually help.

Unfortunately, the biggest obstacle to getting the word out is that these secrets don't make money for the drug companies, doctors or big corporations. Most of them are free or cost very little money. Breast cancer is big business. Breast health is not.

To date, we have spent billions of dollars on research and treatment since the "war on cancer" began. Yet breast cancer is still a threat that countless women face and fear every day. Obviously, there is some-thing missing.

Scientists, the medical community and even the drug companies claim that breast cancer is a very complex problem with no single solution. What they are currently recommending for breast health is what they see as the best answer for women. However, it would appear that while it is putting money in their coffers, it isn't keeping women's breasts healthy and where they belong—on their chests! The global statistics on breast health are solid proof of that.

Women, too, have contributed to this situation. Reluctant to assume responsibility for their breast health, many are much more inclined to turn their breasts over to the medical system. As long as you believe that everyone else has your highest and best interests at heart, you are not only fooling yourself by putting the blinders on, but are actually putting your breast health in a very precarious position.

Complicating matters further is the fact that women are NOT being given critical information that would help them to have healthier breasts. Healthy breasts, just like any other organ of the body, don't get cancer or other debilitating diseases. Most women don't really understand what their breasts need to stay healthy, and breast health is rarely a priority until the word cancer is connected to them.

Part of the reason for this lack of interest and responsibility in breast health is that women are usually excluded from any active participation in their own breast health. There is little to no emphasis placed on breast health and breast cancer prevention through diet, exercise, stress management or regular breast massage. Breasts are more than sexual objects of pleasure for men or a nutritional source of food for babies. They are beautiful, sacred and precious. We need to protect them, love them and cherish them. We need to learn how to take care of them.

So what can you do to educate and protect yourself? In this book, I present to you 21 secrets that you can put into action, today, to increase your breast health. What is so amazing is that many of these are simple, and the majority of them are free or very affordable. Yes, they will require a few changes in your life, but staring breast cancer in the face would require a major change, as any woman or man with breast cancer will attest to.

I want to see you with happy, healthy breasts, so you never have to hear the two words "breast" and "cancer" together in one sentence. I believe that is totally possible. These 21 secrets are a fabulous place to start.

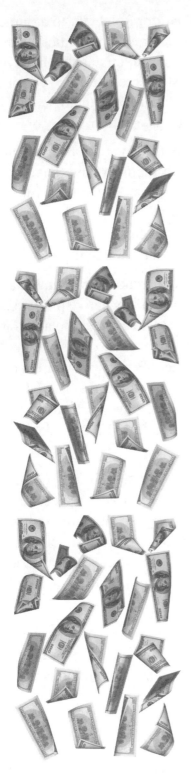

A woman with
breast cancer is worth
between $800,000
and $1.2 million
to the American
medical system.

A woman with
healthy breasts
makes no one
any money!

Secret #1:

Avoid Root Canals

Who would have thought that what goes on in your mouth can seriously affect your breasts? They seem at opposite ends of the health spectrum. When I had a root canal in 2009, I never thought to check out whether or not the procedure was good for me, and it certainly didn't enter my mind that the root canal would affect my breasts. I assumed, as there are 24 million root canals done in the U.S. alone each year, they must be safe. Not true! I wish I had this information then, that I am now sharing with you in this book.

A root canal removes dead or infected nerves and tissue by drilling a hole in the tooth. The root canal area is then cleaned, sterilized and disinfected. The hole is filled and is typically sealed with a crown. The problem is that it is **impossible** to clean out all of the dead tissue or to completely sterilize the tooth. We are talking about 3 miles of tiny channels in every tooth and that is impossible to completely disinfect.

So what's the big deal, as your mouth is constantly full of bacteria anyways, isn't it? The difference is that the dead tissue in the tooth continues to decompose and remains infected. Unlike other areas where the immune system's white blood cells go after the infection, they don't travel into the tiny channels. Hence these tiny channels become breeding grounds for microbes, which include viruses, yeasts, fungi, molds, and bacteria, which are now all stuck in a dead tooth.

Within that dead tooth, there is no oxygen, but bacteria can live without oxygen. Not only does it survive, it mutates in the absence of oxygen into something called thioethers, some of the strongest poisons on the planet.

These thioethers leak into the rest of your body and damage the mitochondria of your cells, causing them to become anaerobic (lacking oxygen). It is very clear that cancer cannot exist in an aerobic environment (one with oxygen) but only in an anaerobic environment, which is exactly what transpires when you have had a root canal.

Dentist Frank Jerome states: "The idea of keeping a dead, infected organ in the body is only thought to be a good idea by dentists. A root canal-treated tooth always negatively affects your immune system."

But what effect do root canals specifically have on your breast health?

"Dr. Thomas Rau, who runs the Paracelsus Clinic (cancer clinic since 1958) in Switzerland recently checked the records of the last 150 breast cancer patients treated in his clinic. He found that 147 of them (98%) had one or more root canal teeth on the same meridian as the original breast cancer tumor. His clinic has a biological dentist section where all cancer patients, on reporting in, have their mouth cleaned up first—especially all root canal teeth removed."

One hundred percent of the breast cancer patients involved in the study had root canals, or other infections, on the same acupuncture meridian. This is not insignificant information when it comes to your overall health, especially your breast health.

Like something out of an old sci-fi movie, dentist Weston Price, back in the 1920's, would take a person who had suffered a heart attack, remove the tooth with the root canal, take a little segment of it, and put it under the skin of a rabbit. In about 10 days, the rabbit would die of a heart attack. If he removed the piece of tooth from the dead rabbit and put it under the skin of another rabbit, in 10 days the second rabbit would die of a heart attack. He would do this to 30 rabbits, and in 97% of the cases, the rabbit would die of heart disease.

In another experiment, Dr. Price removed an infected tooth from a woman who suffered from severe arthritis. He implanted the tooth beneath the skin of a healthy rabbit. Within 48 hours the rabbit was crippled with arthritis.

Dr. Price wrote over 1,100 pages of studies about root canals, much of which is contained in a book called *Root Canal Cover-Up* by Dr. George Meinig, one of the 19 founders of the Association of Endo-dontists and a dentist who performed thousands of root canals over his long career. It wasn't until his retirement that he took the time to read Dr. Price's work from the 1920's and was shocked at the important information and quality studies that had been withheld from public knowledge.

Joseph Issels in Germany treated terminal cancer cases for 40 years. Patients came to Dr. Issels after they already had their chemo, surgery, and radiation treatments and were given less than a year to live. Despite getting his patients when they were in a weakened condition, he turned around 24% of 16,000 patients over a period of 40 years. What is the first thing he did? He had a dentist take out the root canal teeth.

Can this really work? Here's an interesting story related by Bill Henderson, Author of *Cancer Free: Your Guide to Gentle, Non-Toxic Healing*: "Olga (not her real name) had been battling breast cancer, which had spread to many other organs, since the early 1990's. In 1989, Olga moved to New Jersey with her two children. Her bout with cancer started about two years after she arrived there. By the time I met Olga by phone, she had tried a wide variety of conventional and alternative treatments for her cancer. Nothing seemed to help.

"During our telephone conversation in February, 2007, I discussed with Olga... the probable cause of her cancer. When I asked her if she had any root canal filled teeth, she reluctantly admitted that she had ELEVEN. I was shocked. Of the many hundreds of cancer patients I had dealt with, I had never heard of anyone with that many root canals.

"Once I described to Olga the toxic load these teeth were putting on her system, she agreed with me that having them extracted by a biological dentist was essential to her recovery from her cancer. Olga...is finally, for the first time in over 20 years, enjoying complete good health. Her cancer is gone and all her tests are completely clean."

Although dentists will tell you root canals are safe, there are sufficient studies to show unequivocally that they are not safe. They are a big money-maker for the dental industry but they are not in your highest and best interests. The truth is that root canal teeth are a serious health issue that is being swept under the carpet by the medical and dental system.

"A root canal-treated tooth always negatively affects your immune system."
–Dr. Frank Jerome

Secret #2:

Wear Your Bra As Little As Possible

Have you ever thought about how much time your breasts spend in a bra? I never did until I read the book *Dressed to Kill: The Link Between Breast Cancer and Bras,* over two years ago. That was when I liberated my breasts and I now rarely wear a bra. I have never had such happy, healthy breasts as I do now that they know freedom.

What made me go from a woman with a bra to match every outfit to the camisole queen I am today? I learned some facts that made me stop and think very seriously about my breast health. Then I proved to myself how uncomfortable bras really are by wearing my bra as little as possible over the last 24 months. We've simply grown accustomed to the discomfort of wearing a bra and have conformed to a cultural standard. However, you may be surprised at the statistics. In a study completed by two medical anthropologists, Sydney Ross Singer and Soma Grismaijer, it was discovered:

- 3 out of 4 women who wore their bras 24 hours per day developed breast cancer.

- 1 out of 7 women who wore bras more than 12 hours per day but not to bed developed breast cancer.

- 1 out of 152 women who wore their bras less than 12 hours per day got breast cancer.

- 1 out of 168 women who rarely or never wore bras got breast cancer.

Women who wear their bra 24 hours a day have a 125-fold (12,500%) higher percentage of getting cancer than women who do not wear a bra at all. There is a six-fold (600%) greater incidence of breast cancer among women who wear a bra all day and to bed than among the general population.

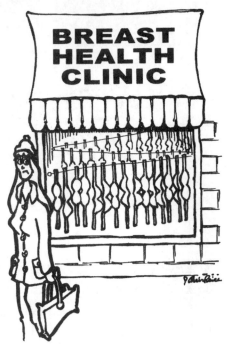

Why are bras potentially not good for you? How many times have you taken off your bra and noticed red marks or indentations either on your shoulders, under your breasts or on your back? You have been trained to believe that this is just the price you pay for being a woman and having to wear a bra. Nobody has ever told you those marks are indicative of something going awry; but in fact, it is your body's way of communicating with you.

Most people are aware of the immune system—the system that keeps us healthy and strong, fights disease and protects us from all sorts of enemies, both externally and internally. The lymphatic system is an important part of that immune system. Lymph fluid flows through your body, cleansing your tissues of toxins. If you have ever taken off a pair of tight-fitting knee highs or shoes, and your feet or legs are swollen, that is a result of a backup of this lymph fluid.

When a toxin enters your body, it gets flushed away by the lymphatic system. But if the lymphatic system is impaired or restricted from entering certain parts of your body, then the toxins enter, but the cleaners can't get in to clean. Imagine a teenager's messy room as a visual. The garbage keeps on coming in but the cleaners are barred from entering. Pretty soon it's a pig sty.

Toxins are entering your body daily in minute amounts. Today, you can't breathe without taking in toxins. The body in its infinite wisdom, deliberately stores toxins in fat cells for safekeeping. However, when too much builds up in one area, cancer or other serious diseases can develop. In women, one of the largest areas of fat is found in breast tissue—this is why breast cancer is so prevalent.

Are you starting to see the problem? Our breasts are full of toxins but the toxins aren't able to get out because the lymphatic system is restricted…by our bras. The toxins then pool, trapped in the cage called a bra, which most women wear every day.

Interestingly, in Korea, they have noticed a massive upswing recently in breast cancer in women. A documentary linked the possible increase to more Korean women wearing Western style clothing, including bras. What was also fascinating in this study was that upwards of 80% of women are wearing their bras 24 hours a day. What has seemed like "the thing to do," as countries mimic a western lifestyle, is proving to be unhealthy.

Dr. Elizabeth R. Vaughan of North Carolina in the U.S. is a strong proponent of going bra-free and has been preaching this message to her patients for over 25 years. She says, "Breasts are loaded with lymphatic tissue. The lymphatic system doesn't have a "pump" like the heart. Movement and massage help move toxins along our lymphatic system. Anything that slows down the clearing of these toxins will increase an individual's risk of developing symptoms and/or disease. Bras, which restrict movement of the breasts, appear to increase congestion in the breasts and slow down clearance of toxins from the breasts, which will increase the rate that women develop breast diseases. Why? Because the toxins remain concentrated in otherwise healthy tissue for much longer."

Bottom line: Breasts need to jiggle. Going braless does not make breasts sag. It actually strengthens the ligaments you have to support your breasts. They've just gotten lazy—similar to what would happen if you put your arm in a sling and never used it.

I get on my rebounder that sits beside my desk several times a day and bounce for a few minutes to get my lymphatic system revved up. I can feel my energy increase and I can go from feeling tired or sluggish to energized in minutes. By going braless, your breasts can begin to experience some of that healthy up and down movement, critical to breast health.

You can cut down on your bra usage by removing it when you are at home and not wearing it at night. When you do wear a bra, ensure that it's not leaving red marks on your shoulders, as this is an indication that your lymphatic system is being compromised. Statistically, most women wear the wrong size of bra; so if you're going to wear a bra, then get it properly fitted so it's as healthy as it can be for your breasts. And it is highly recommended by doctors, such as Dr. Christine Northrup, that women don't wear underwire bras.

This is a shift for most women, as we have been taught that we need to cover up our breasts, and there is something wrong or bad if our nipples show. We need to get over that for the sake of our health. Breasts are literally screaming for help, as they are desperately trying to fight off the toxins while having all exit ways blocked. Many breasts are losing the battle and succumbing to diseases such as cancer.

So let your breasts experience freedom as much as possible. They will thank you for it!

Remember...

◆ Take off your bra as much as possible when you don't need to wear it (i.e. at home and definitely at night).

◆ Get a properly fitted bra that doesn't leave red marks!

Secret #3:

Get Your Lymphatic System Moving

While the topic of your lymphatic system is fresh in your mind, let's discuss another secret that can help reduce breast pain and help you have happy, healthy breasts.

Lymphatic massage helps the flow of lymph in your breast tissue and as you just read, that lymph fluid gets stuck and can stagnate. A quick five-minute massage can help your breasts feel better and it's easy.

Many women experience breast lumps that are not cancerous, but are actually full of this lymph fluid. Get the fluid moving with massage and lumps, and other breast pain or discomfort can vanish.

By increasing circulation and promoting lymphatic drainage, your breasts will feel better (less or no lumps), feel lighter, and be pain-free.

In addition to non-specific gentle massage of the breasts, there are massage techniques that have been devised to be more efficient in promoting lymph drainage of breast tissue. If you have any breast-related medical conditions, consult your physician prior to initiating any regular self-massage program. The best way to learn how to do lymphatic breast massage is by watching someone teach you. Reading how to do it is much more challenging and with this easy 5-minute video you can follow along as you do your own breast massage.

http://breasthealthrevolution.com/resources/videos/

Breathing deeply massages your lymphatic trunk, increasing lymph circulation. Daya Fisch, breast health expert (and the instructor on the video) suggests that we learn to breathe better. Instead of feeling your stress levels rise every time you find yourself waiting, like in the long grocery store line or the dentist's office, why don't you do some deep breathing your breasts will love you for.

See all those yucky toxins making their way out of your breasts and being eliminated through your lymphatic system. Here's an easy deep breathing technique your breasts will love. Put your hands on your belly, take ten deep slow breaths. Feel your belly rise and fall. As you breathe out, push the air out of your lungs. Use your stomach muscles and tighten your rib cage to get all the air out. The "in" breath happens easily and naturally. Fill your whole chest and belly with air. Repeat this process. There is no need to hold your breath, just breathe easily and rhythmically. Imagine breathing beauty, wellness or love into your being. Feel your body draw nourishment from the breath.

To go faster, (after you are comfortable with the slow breathing) start slow and speed up. Push the air out of your body using the stomach muscles. This breath takes longer to become comfortable. Start slow. Begin with five fast breaths, then ten, and build up your strength. You could work up to a full minute. It is great and you will feel very energized! If you feel dizzy, stop. And please, don't do this fast deep breathing while you drive. After you breathe, sit quietly for a few seconds.

Once you get comfortable with breathing, imagine that it is not just oxygen coming into your body, but nourishing, loving energy. Call it Life force, Chi, Prana, Spirit, Love—or whatever name you choose to use.

Here's the third tip to get your lymphatic system moving that's easy and feels fabulous. I personally do dry brushing every day before jumping in the shower. By using a long-handled brush, I spend about two minutes in this very enjoyable activity, which starts my day off.

Dry Skin Brushing Routine

- Purchase a natural bristle brush (usually made for skin brushing) from a natural or whole foods market.

- Keep your brush dry at all times.

- Brush in short, light, upward strokes. These can get more firm as your skin gets used to brushing.

- Brush your whole body every day from the feet up, always toward your heart.

- Brush the bottom of your left foot first, then ankle, calf and thigh. Repeat on your right foot and leg.

- Brush your buttocks and front of hips then your stomach, circling around your navel.

- Brush up your torso and around breasts toward heart – do not brush your nipples.

- Brush your hands up each arm toward your heart.

- Brush from your chin down your neck and chest toward your heart.

- The entire routine should only take from 2-4 minutes each day.

- An added benefit would be to take a warm shower afterward and end with cool water. This also stimulates your lymph drainage.

Each month, take a week's break from dry-brushing, especially if you're brushing daily. This keeps the body from becoming overly habituated to the practice, ensuring maximum benefit from it during your active periods.

Never share your brush; each family member should have her or his own. Wash your brush or mitt every couple of weeks in warm water using a mild soap and hang it to dry in an area that allows air circulation on all sides to prevent the growth of mildew.

By taking a few minutes each week to clear the toxins out of your breasts through lymphatic stimulation with massage, deep breathing and dry brushing, your breasts can stay healthier, happier and much safer. Especially if you have lumpy breasts or painful breasts, this is a big clue that your breasts inside look more like a garbage dump than a pristine meadow. You're worth this extra pampering and your breasts will so appreciate the tender loving care.

Helpful Hint:

A professional lymphatic massage can be the answer to getting your lymphatic system moving. Just be sure you choose someone properly trained and with lots of experience!

Secret #4:

Sweat it Out

We are a society committed to smelling pretty and pretending we don't perspire. But our obsession with stopping underarm perspiration may also be killing us.

Deodorant, unlike antiperspirant, does not block the release of underarm perspiration. It neutralizes the smell, using antiseptic ingredients that deal with the bacteria. Antiperspirants actually clog or block the pores that release sweat.

Your body needs to release toxins. However, when you use an antiperspirant, you stop a key area of detoxification. The toxins—meant to be expelled through the underarms—get deposited in the lymph nodes below the arms.

Studies have continually shown that nearly all breast cancers occur in the upper outer quadrant (UOQ) of the breast. Interestingly, this is precisely where the lymph nodes are located!

The proportion of breast cancer in the UOQ of the breast has been rising steadily with the increased use of antiperspirants and deodorants. In 1926, 31% of breast cancers occurred in the UOQ; in 1947-1967 this percentage increased to 43-48%. Currently about 62% of breast cancers occur in the part of the breast that is the closest to the armpit.

However, this topic is as controversial as whether or not wearing bras is actually bad for you. Bra manufacturers will tell you there is no danger in wearing bras, just as the Cosmetic and Toiletry industry will tell you there is no correlation between antiperspirants and breast cancer. However, evidence proves otherwise—in both cases.

Let's start with what's in antiperspirants and deodorants. They all contain aluminum in some form.

The *Journal of Inorganic Biochemistry* states: "We have confirmed the presence of aluminum in breast tissue… Higher content of aluminum in the outer breast might be explained by this region's closer proximity to the underarm where the highest density of application of antiperspirant could be assumed. There is evidence that skin is permeable to aluminum when applied as antiperspirant."

After a single underarm application of antiperspirant, about .012 percent of the aluminum may be absorbed. That may seem miniscule, but considering that most people apply deodorant at least once per day 365 days a year for most of their lives, it adds up.

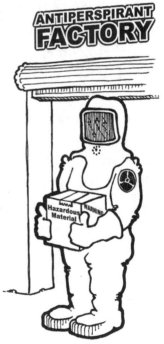

A 2001 study showed that aluminum was still present in blood samples 15 days after one application of aluminum to the armpit, so it obviously doesn't dissipate quickly.

But is aluminum dangerous? One document outlining safety protocol for a deodorant factory has serious warnings about inhalation and skin contact. Protective clothing included a vented hood, gloves, lab coat and goggles —all mandatory. Just think about this. The employees who work with aluminum need to protect themselves from this hazardous material, yet we put it on our underarms and are being assured it's safe. A rather interesting thought, wouldn't you agree?

Because you are accustomed to using aluminum foil or aluminum cookware in food preparation, you may not think of aluminum as toxic, but it is.

Aluminum was first recognized as a human neurotoxin—a substance that causes damage to nerves or nerve tissue—way back in 1886. It has been well established that the accumulation of aluminum in the brain can cause neurological disorders, with even the World Health Organization back in 1993 admitting that "there is a suspected link between Alzheimer's disease and the toxicity of aluminum." But what about breast health?

In 2004, Dr. Kris McGrath, a Chicago allergist, performed a study published in the *European Journal of Cancer Prevention* which found a connection between antiperspirants, underarm shaving, and cancer. He studied 400 Chicago-area breast cancer survivors and found that women *"who performed these underarm habits more aggressively"* had a diagnosis of breast cancer twenty-two years earlier than the non-users. Dr. McGrath theorized that substances found in deodorants, such as aluminum chlorohydrate, were entering the lymphatic system through nicks in the skin caused by shaving.

Most deodorants contain aluminum zirconium, which is toxic to the nervous and reproductive systems, and a chemical called BHT, which is included in the list of endocrine disrupting chemicals. This means it affects the reproductive system, including the sex hormones, which is what contributes to breast cancer.

And if you use a spray deodorant, you are being subjected to propellants such as butane, isobutene, and propane, which sound more like a barbeque lighter fluid than something you want on your body. PPG-14 Butyl ether, the preservative solvent used in deodorant sprays, is potentially toxic to the kidneys and liver. The liver is critical to every aspect of your health but particularly your hormonal health. PPG-14 Butyl ether is also a pesticide component used in sprays to protect animals from flies and mosquitoes. It hardly sounds appropriate for human use.

And then there is the better-known issue of parabens, which are found in deodorants. Researchers have found traces of chemicals called parabens in every sample of tissue taken from 20 different breast tumors. Parabens have been shown to be able to mimic the action of the female hormone estrogen, which can drive the growth of human breast tumors.

The other primary ingredient in deodorants is fragrance. However, the whole world of fragrances, including perfumes, colognes, shampoos, AND deodorants, is completely unregulated. The Federal Fair Packaging and Labeling Act of 1973 explicitly exempts fragrance as one ingredient that does not need to be disclosed. However, many of the ingredients in fragrances are substances that have never been assessed for safety in personal care products. Many of these chemicals are associated with hormone disruption.

For example, diethyl phthalate, a chemical found in 97 percent of Americans, is linked to sperm damage. Musk ketone, another synthetic fragrance ingredient concentrates in human fat tissue and breast milk. A pregnant woman is rarely, if ever, admonished to avoid perfumes and toxic cosmetic products, yet her unborn fetus is getting the brunt of these potent chemicals that are dangerous and are largely untested.

So in deodorants and antiperspirants, we have aluminum, which leads to neurological damage and is a hazardous material, we have parabens that mimic estrogen and are endocrine disruptors, and fragrance ingredients that are unregulated. Makes you want to go and put on some deodorant right now, doesn't it? But what about the smell?

Obviously no one wants to go around with body odor. However, body odor is your body's way of letting you know that something rotten is going on inside. There is putrefaction and decay happening, and body odor manifesting on the outside is a symptom of what is occurring within your body.

A diet that relies primarily on red meat, processed foods and sugar, will emit a totally different odor than one that is more plant-based and focuses on unrefined foods.

Achieving a more pleasant body odor naturally is another great reason to make sure that your elimination processes such as your lymphatic system and your bowels are working effectively.

There are some deodorants available that are safe and don't contain aluminum, synthetic fragrances or parabens. Check out the store at www.breasthealthrevolution.com for my latest recommendation. In the meantime, you might just want to sweat it out!

Secret #5:

Get Out in the Sunshine

Perhaps you have heard that we're vitamin D deficient. Recent studies are showing than more than 75% of the population either has insufficient or deficient levels of vitamin D. How is this important vitamin linked to your breast health?

In a vitamin D conference held in Toronto, Canada in November 2009, Dr. Cedric Garland stated: "Breast cancer is a disease so directly related to vitamin D deficiency that a woman's risk of contracting the disease can be **'virtually eradicated'** by elevating her vitamin D status to what vitamin D scientists consider to be natural blood levels."

Wow! That is a powerful statement. Could it really be that easy to protect your breasts by simply getting more vitamin D in your body?

Thirty of the world's leading researchers on vitamin D recommend 2,000 IU of vitamin D daily (up substantially from the current 400 IU) and vitamin D blood levels of 100-150 nanomoles-per-liter as measured by a vitamin D blood test.

Garland, whose presentation was entitled "Breast Cancer as a Vitamin D Deficiency Disease" presented data showing that raising one's vitamin D status near those levels decreased breast cancer risk more than 77 percent.

Dr. Mercola explains that each cell in your body has its own 'DNA library' that contains information needed to deal with virtually every kind of stimulus it may encounter, and **the master key to enter this library is activated vitamin D.**

For example, memory ductile cells in a woman's breasts need vitamin D to access DNA that enables the response to estrogen.

So it stands to reason that without sufficient amounts of vitamin D, your cells cannot access their DNA libraries. As a result, their functions are impaired and all sorts of problems can ensue, depending on how well your cells are able to compensate for the lack of vitamin D.

Facts about Vitamin D:

1. The vast majority of the western population is deficient in vitamin D.

2. Vitamin D deficiencies promote cancer, diabetes, osteoporosis, kidney disease, depression, obesity and heart disease, among other health problems.

3. Vitamin D deficiencies can be corrected with vitamin D supplementation or through sensible sunlight exposure.

4. Sunscreen products *block the production* of vitamin D in the skin, causing further vitamin D deficiencies across the population of consumers who use such products.

5. Correcting widespread vitamin D deficiencies would greatly reduce degenerative disease across the population, thereby saving nations literally *trillions* of dollars in collective sick-care costs over the next decade.

6. Vitamin D supplements are extremely affordable. Preventing disease through vitamin D supplementation is a low-cost investment in health that pays off a hundred fold (or more) through health care cost savings.

7. Vitamin D is extremely safe. There are virtually no negative side effects from deficient people taking vitamin D supplements, even at seemingly high doses such as 4000 - 8000 IU per day (more than ten times the current U.S. RDA).

8. Vitamin D deficiency is caused, in large part, by modern society's **indoor lifestyle**. People live, work and play indoors under artificial light. This causes severe deficiencies in exposure to *natural light* (sunlight) through which vitamin D is usually generated.

9. Vitamin D dramatically reduces susceptibility to infectious disease such as seasonal flu and H1N1. It "activates" the immune system and allows it to function more aggressively in defending against viral invasions.

Where do you get vitamin D? The body can make its own vitamin D following exposure to UVB radiation from the sun. Adequate exposure typically requires around 15 to 20 minutes of midday sunlight, two to three times per week. However, thanks to the brainwashing by the media and the medical system, people today aren't getting out in the sun and certainly they aren't venturing outside without toxic sunscreen slathered on.

Two problems come about as a result:

1. This particular ultraviolet light is not available during the winter months at some latitudes. The greater the distance from the equator, the less UVB there is.

2. We need to actually expose ourselves to sunshine—without sunscreen. What a novel concept!

There are also dietary sources of vitamin D, but it's practically impossible to get enough from food alone. Some examples include fatty fish such as salmon, egg yolks and fortified milk. To reach even bare minimum levels would require drinking around 20 glasses of milk every single day. Not a practical solution!

Yet, studies show that 8 out of 10 cancers could be prevented with sufficient vitamin D. Why aren't you told about this critically important nutrient in your pursuit of breast health? The medical system, which is closely aligned with the pharmaceutical companies, cannot regulate or monetize vitamin D from sunshine. Unless they can make money on it, they will keep you in the dark—literally! As little as 10 to 20 minutes a day of sunshine on your unprotected body can make a difference to your health.

Get yourself tested for your vitamin D level. To find out exactly what to look for, visit www.breasthealthrevolution.com/resources/medicaltests where you will find information from health expert Dr. Mercola on what to look for in vitamin D testing.

If there was any doubt about the importance of vitamin D for your breast health, just note the areas where there is the most breast cancer. The states with the least sunlight (Oregon and Washington on the West Coast, far Northern states like Minnesota and Eastern seaboard states) have the highest rates of breast cancer. Meanwhile, virtually all the states along the sunbelt (Arizona, New Mexico, Texas, Alabama, Florida, etc.) have the lowest rates of breast cancer.

"Breast cancer is a disease directly related to vitamin D deficiency"
–Dr. Cedric Garland

Ninety-seven percent of Canadians are deficient in vitamin D because of their northern exposure; and as a Canadian who loves her sunshine, I can attest to that!

Another study released in 2008 found that women with breast cancer and low levels of vitamin D may have a poorer prognosis than those with sufficient vitamin D. The study by Toronto researchers also found that women with too little of the vitamin had a greater chance of recurrence and lower overall survival rates than those with healthier amounts.

The study involved 512 women, aged 35 to 69, who were diagnosed with breast cancer between 1989 and 1996. Their health was followed until 2007, on average for almost 12 years. The researchers found that 37.5 percent of the patients were vitamin D deficient and 38.5 percent had levels that were considered insufficient for good bone health. Only 24 per cent had sufficient levels of vitamin D in their blood.

Are you ready to bring more sunshine into your life? Vitamin D is an important piece of the breast health puzzle that is missing today. So get your vitamin D levels up to where they need to be for optimal health and see how much different you feel!

Secret #6:

Sleep in the Dark

Sleep is one of the most challenging things today. Over 40% of the population has interrupted sleep at night. If you have tossed and turned all night, woken up in the middle of the night and not been able to go back to sleep, or have experienced long-term insomnia, you know how important sleep is. However, it's even more important than you may have realized when it comes to your breast health.

At night your body produces a hormone called melatonin. Secreted by the pineal gland in the brain, it is mostly dormant during the day. It then gets switched on at about 9 p.m. and shuts down around 9 a.m. The peak hours of operation are between 2 and 4 in the morning. Melatonin makes you feel sleepy, less alert and is what keeps you asleep.

Melatonin is called the "dark" hormone and is only made after your body has been exposed to very bright light in the day and then complete darkness at night. You can see why getting a dose of sunshine in the day can help you sleep better at night. But there's an important caveat to the production of melatonin.

It needs to be dark when you sleep. That means no street lights shining into your bedroom, no night lights, bright alarm clocks and no lights shining off of electronic equipment such as TVs, or DVDs. Total darkness is needed to produce optimal levels of melatonin.

If sleeping in a dark room is impossible because of traveling or a partner who needs a nightlight for night trips to the bathroom, then you can use a mask to cover your eyes. This will take a few nights to get used to but is very effective at creating a dark atmosphere.

If you get up to go to the bathroom at night and turn on the light, your melatonin production stops for the entire night. It doesn't restart once you turn off the light. This interruption has been clearly shown to dramatically increase your risk of most cancers, but especially breast and prostate cancers.

Melatonin also helps control the timing and release of female reproductive hormones, including estrogen. It helps determine when a woman starts to menstruate, the frequency and duration of menstrual cycles, and when a woman stops menstruating (menopause). It is because of this strong link to your hormones, including estrogen, that it is an important element to you having healthy breasts.

Several studies have suggested that melatonin levels may be associated with breast cancer risk. For example, women with breast cancer tend to have lower levels of melatonin than those without the disease. Laboratory experiments have found that low levels of melatonin stimulate the growth of certain types of breast cancer cells, while adding melatonin to these cells slows their growth.

David E. Blask, MD, PhD and an expert in melatonin and cancer, reported that melatonin puts breast cancer cells to sleep, and it also slows breast cancer growth by 70%. When lab mice with human breast cancers were exposed to constant light: **tumor growth skyrocketed**. Eva S. Schernhammer and her Harvard colleague Susan E. Hankinson found that women who happen to have above-average melatonin concentrations are relatively unlikely to develop breast cancer. "Those with higher levels seem to have lower breast cancer risk," said Schernhammer.

It has also been found that totally blind women had a 36% lower risk of breast cancer compared with sighted women. Women who became blind relatively early in life (before age 65) appeared to be especially protected against breast cancer, with incidence rates 49% below those of sighted women.

Only total blindness—not visual impairment—seems to protect against breast cancer. According to the study, this supports the theory that increased nighttime exposure to artificial light reduces melatonin levels, altering estrogen secretion rates and upping risks for breast cancer.

The increased risk of breast cancer seen in flight attendants and shift or night workers may be due to disruption of sleep-wake cycles and a consequent reduction in melatonin production.

There are factors that will decrease or stop melatonin production and these are important to avoid if you are having a difficult time sleeping and staying asleep.

- Caffeine

- Tobacco

- Alcohol (may get you to sleep but wakes you up in the night)

- Chocolate (especially dark)

- Aspirin, Tylenol

- Most anti-depressants like Prozac and sleep medications (all promote shallow, not deep sleep)

- Being close to electrical appliances (within 3 feet) especially electric blankets

What does all of this mean for you and your breasts?

1. Take getting enough sleep seriously – 7 to 9 hours every night.

2. Sleep in the dark so you have optimum melatonin production.

3. Be exposed to bright light every day, either naturally or through appropriate artificial lighting sources.

4. Avoid the enemies of melatonin as much as possible in your diet.

5. If you're not sleeping well, consider a melatonin supplement after checking in with your health care practitioner.

I find that if I am tossing and turning at night, a melatonin supplement
will ensure a good night's sleep so that is always an option and a very
affordable one.

Now that you understand the importance of melatonin in your body,
commit to a good night's sleep....in the dark. Your whole body will
thank you for this one!

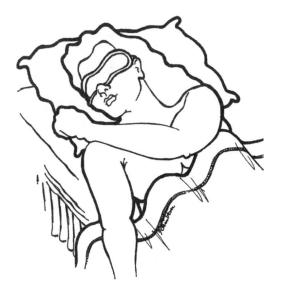

Secret #7:

Find Ways to Deal with Stress

W ho doesn't know the meaning of stress these days? Every person on the planet, including children and the elderly are feeling the effects of stress. So it is completely unreasonable to think we can live stress-free, but there are important things we can do to reduce stress and deal better with it.

Why is this important for your breast health? This is actually a two-pronged question and answer.

We have become inundated with frightening facts and scary statistics about breast cancer to the point that every woman lives with that fear either consciously or subconsciously affecting her body. This is neither healthy nor desirable. By learning more about your breasts and empowering yourself with knowledge and taking small steps towards healthier breasts, you can actually relieve some of that stress that is being hammered home daily by the media and the medical system.

By understanding that every day your body deals with viruses, bacteria and cancer and **wins the battle daily**, rather than obsess and get stressed out worrying about cancer, why not focus on the marvelous job your body is either doing or is capable of doing? Just that simple shift in perspective can relieve you of some stress. Empower your body to deal with cancer and bring your body into better health daily.

Seriously, most people die with cancer in their bodies, even if it was never detected in their lifetime. Autopsies have proven this. Dr. Ben Johnson, the well-known oncologist from the movie *The Secret,* states that most women over 50 have DCIS (ductal carcinoma in situ), a tiny cancer that is in the milk ducts of the breasts. In other words, we have become obsessed with cancer, which we all have to some degree or another, instead of focusing on health.

Dr. Welch, author of *Should I be Tested for Cancer* concludes his book with these words: "Pursuing disease is not at all the same as pursuing health. In fact, they easily conflict. It can be quite difficult to promote wellness when you are actively looking for things to be wrong."

Dr. Ben Johnson says, "Obsessing with fear about getting breast cancer sends an unhealthy message to the cells, where it becomes implanted in your cellular memory."

Top holistic doctor, Norm Shealy, links cancer to depression, and Dr. Ryke Geerd Hamer links breast cancer to emotional upsets, trauma and/or shock. Stanford University Scientist Dr. Bruce Lipton's research shows that chronic stress is responsible for 95% of all diseases.

So first relieve yourself of the stress around breast cancer by focusing on your empowerment and knowledge in the arena of breast health! It is much easier to have healthy breasts than you have been led to believe.

Secondly, let's deal with the stress. If your shoulders and earlobes are practically touching or you are grinding your teeth, not sleeping well or suffering from other symptoms of chronic stress.....learn to chill!

What can chilling look like? For some it's meditation, yoga or qigong, tai chi or some other Eastern practice. I love to go for a brisk walk in the sun, spend an evening with friends playing Yahtzee or cards or curl up with a good mystery novel. I also daily jump on a rebounder and take out some of my tension bouncing on the mini-trampoline.

Does having a hot bath with candlelight and a good book do it for you? When was the last time you had a day off and did something you wanted to do? If you can't remember, that's a big clue that you need to take this chapter very seriously.

A University of Pittsburgh study actually showed that people who go to church every week add an average of three years to their lives. I believe that a strong spiritual connection, however that looks for you, can indeed be an aid to releasing stress.

Women can be real martyrs when it comes to looking after everybody else. The problem with that complex is that it comes back to bite you….hard. What happens when you find yourself with something seriously wrong so you can't look after anybody, not even yourself?

If you're skipping through this chapter with the idea in your mind, "yeah well I can't get rid of my stress because of…." or are looking for that magic pill to deal with your stress, stop and know that I am especially speaking to you! The body has an amazing way of making you deal with your excess stress. It's called disease. And you are more susceptible to disease if you aren't listening to your body's communication with you.

Dr. Nan Lu, a traditional Chinese doctor, comments in his book, *A Woman's Guide to Healing from Breast Cancer,* that many women wear like a badge of honor that they are right back to the level of activity where they were before their diagnosis of breast cancer and can even be congratulated by others for re-achieving that insane level of stress. However, if that's a contributing factor to what created a problem in the first place, why would you go back there?

According to Traditional Chinese Medicine which has been practiced for over 5,000 years, worry is related to the spleen. If you always worry or continually over-think, you will cause stomach and spleen Qi (pronounced chee) stagnation. In this case, you might lose your appetite, have digestive system problems, retain water, or find it difficult to lose weight. Interestingly, more than 50% of breast cancers are diagnosed in the area of the breast where your stomach meridians run.

Dr. Lu says, "All female problems—either directly or indirectly, relate to liver function. When liver function is poor, your Qi and blood can stagnate. It is precisely this stagnation, over time, that can lead to the formation of masses and tumors. Liver stagnation is caused by anger and over-thinking. Poor liver function can show up in anger, depression, stress, or uneven moods, frustration, irritability, or nervous tension. Stress goes right to your liver where it can either cause or aggravate many problems."

We all know that too much stress isn't good for us. It doesn't take a rocket scientist or a medical doctor to tell us that. But most of us don't listen until something serious happens like depression, chronic fatigue or cancer. That's just not smart as I am sure you would agree. There is a better way.

Do something now to relieve the stress before your body gets really serious about letting you know you need to relax.

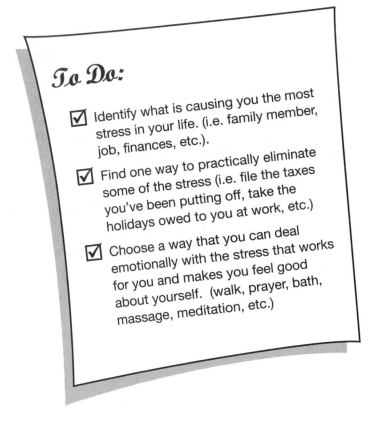

To Do:

☑ Identify what is causing you the most stress in your life. (i.e. family member, job, finances, etc.).

☑ Find one way to practically eliminate some of the stress (i.e. file the taxes you've been putting off, take the holidays owed to you at work, etc.)

☑ Choose a way that you can deal emotionally with the stress that works for you and makes you feel good about yourself. (walk, prayer, bath, massage, meditation, etc.)

Secret #8:

Wash All New Clothes Before You Wear Them

Clothing today is very toxic. Non-organic clothing contains residues of pesticides, formaldehyde, chlorine, fire retardant and synthetic chemical dyes. Chemical residues from the cloth, along with the chemicals from the detergents used to wash it, are absorbed through the skin throughout the day.

Our skin is the largest organ in the body that readily absorbs the toxic chemicals that it comes into contact with. If you don't believe that fact, just think of the nicotine patch, the motion sickness patch and the birth control patch. They work because the moisture on our skin acts as a conductor and allows chemicals to be absorbed.

Unless you are a nudist, you are either wearing clothes or are in bed against sheets, which are usually toxic. In other words, your body is dealing with toxic chemicals right up close and personal with your skin, 24 hours a day.

Many of these toxins have been linked to numerous health problems including allergies, insomnia, immune disorders, cancer, and more.

I know that I love the feel of cotton, so I try to buy it as much as possible. Cotton T-shirts are cheap; and up until recently, I thought were the healthiest for my body. Not necessarily so.

It requires almost the entire weight of a cotton t-shirt in fertilizers and pesticides to grow the cotton for it. That's right. Cotton uses only 2.4% of the world's agricultural acreage, however its cultivation involves

25% of the world's pesticide use, and it accounts for 11% of global pesticide sales.

Cotton is the most pesticide-intensive crop grown on the planet. Of the most commonly used pesticides, seven of them are suspected or known to be carcinogens (causing cancer). Non-organic cotton is one of the most environmentally destructive crops to grow. In California, five of the top nine pesticides used on cotton are cancer-causing chemicals.

Several washings are done throughout the entire process, but some of the softeners and detergents leave a residue that will not totally be removed from the final product. Chemicals often used for finishing include formaldehyde, caustic soda, sulfuric acid, bromines, urea resins, sulfonamides, halogens, and bromines. Non-organic cotton cloth in clothing is bleached and chemically dyed before being treated with formaldehyde, which is known to cause respiratory disorders and insomnia. Additional chemicals are used to resist shrinking and wrinkling and to make it more resistant to fire. All of these chemical residues are absorbed by the skin.

That simple little cotton T-shirt blended with polyester can release approximately one quarter of its weight in air pollutants and 10 times its weight in carbon dioxide. That cotton T-shirt doesn't feel quite as healthy or good for the planet any longer, does it?

Demand for man-made fibers such as petroleum-derived polyester has nearly doubled in the last 15 years. "The manufacturing of polyester and other synthetic fabrics is an energy-intensive process requiring large amounts of crude oil. The processes emit volatile organic compounds and solvents, particulate matter, acid gases such as hydrogen chloride, and other production by-products into the air and water."

In developing countries, where most clothing today is made, regulations are less stringent. The amount of herbicides and insecticides used, and their toxicity, is often greater than in the U.S. Of the 216 chemicals that induced breast tumors in lab animals, humans are "highly exposed" to 97 of them.

And what about your bra, which is right up against your breasts, sometimes for several hours each day? They too contain carcinogenic chemicals that need to be removed as much as possible before the first wearing. There are very easy ways to remove at least some of the chemicals.

What can you do that will help protect your breasts?

1. Whenever possible, purchase clothing made from organic materials, especially cotton. Hemp is another great alternative and is becoming more popular. Organic wool and linen are other options.

2. Use non-toxic laundry soap in your laundry. Otherwise you are adding to the chemicals, not taking away. A cup of vinegar in the laundry has been touted as doing lots of good things including removing odors and some of the chemicals.

3. Don't use dryer sheets as they are full of all sorts of toxic chemicals including Benzyl Acetate, Benzyl Alcohol, Chloroform and Linalool; none of which are good for the environment—or you. Some of these compounds are known carcinogens. There are natural alternatives to dryer sheets, such as using non-PVC dryer balls or adding baking soda to the final rinse.

4. Wash all clothing before you wear them. And if clothes smell particularly toxic (they are now applying a long-lasting disinfectant to some clothes), it's probably best to not even buy them.

Hopefully, you are beginning to see that breast health is a series of little things that can add up to big changes overall. There is no one cause of breast cancer, so there isn't going to be one solution either. However, by making small changes, we can have healthier breasts …and a whole lot healthier planet as a side benefit.

The Sobering Facts

- Seventeen different types of pesticide were found in a woman's breast tissue.

- Women eliminate 40-50% of their accumulated harmful toxins during their first pregnancies.

- Fire retardant showed up 10-20 times higher in breast milk in the U.S. than in Europe, where these chemicals are being phased out.

- Women with breast cancer have 50-60 percent more pesticides in their breast tissue than women without breast cancer.

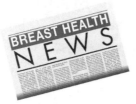

The Good News

- You can use natural products, save yourself money, and heal the planet.

- There are many easy ways to keep your breasts healthy that you can do yourself!

- By detoxifying your breasts BEFORE you get pregnant, you can reduce the toxic load transferred to your baby!

See www.breasthealthrevolution.com
for more great ideas!

Secret #9:

Take Breast Health Back Into Your Own Hands

Many women are probably expecting this secret to be all about breast self-exams (BSE) and you may already be cringing at the thought of having to commit to a monthly exam. I assure you, there is much more to taking breast health back into your own hands than looking for cancer every month.

But let's start there—and put your mind at ease. Although 90% of lumps are found by women, most women don't do the monthly self-exam. Afraid to find cancer, it feels like one of those times when you'd rather not know. The element of fear is huge and can overwhelm any sense that it would be wise to get to know your breasts.

I've felt that fear also. I think every woman has. I agree that scheduling time each month to look for cancer is not the mindset or attitude to achieve optimum breast health. It's why I much prefer what Dr. Nan Lu, author of *Traditional Chinese Medicine: A Woman's Guide to Healing from Breast Cancer,* has to say about breast self-exams.

He says: "Monthly BSE can be approached as an energy healing experience. Instead of worrying about where the cancer might be located, I recommend telling yourself instead that wherever you touch, you are sending in healing energy to protect that location so you will never have breast cancer." Then he suggests that you have whatever tests you choose as confirmation that your own prevention program is working.

As long as you are afraid to touch your breasts or get to know them intimately, they will remain strangers. It is one of the reasons that twice daily, I massage my breasts with Dr. Spencer's Breast Cream. This is a beautiful breast cream designed by a medical doctor. With the primary ingredient being spirulina algae, one of the most powerful detoxifiers on the planet, it feels like a good thing to do for my breasts, because my breasts are inevitably full of environmental toxins.

It also gives me opportunity to be in touch with my breasts daily and to notice anything untoward. I don't go looking for problems but focus on loving my breasts and affirming their place on my body and in my life. "The girls" are staying right where they are, thank you very much, and I remind them of that daily.

Many women use the Plexus Breast Chek Kit, which acts as a magnifier for your fingertips and will find lumps long before they would be palpable using just your fingers. This product has been used by doctors all over the world, is registered with the FDA, and has been touted as finding lumps earlier than a clinical breast exam or even mammography. It makes looking for any irregularity so much easier than just the pads of your fingers. One of my dearest friends helped her elderly mother find breast cancer using this specially designed pad over eight years ago. Her mom just passed away at 93, her breast cancer a long forgotten problem.

Many cancer organizations have downplayed the role each woman can have in her own breast health. They've even discouraged BSE and admonished women that an annual mammogram is sufficient. However, many disagree with that ever-changing point of view.

According to Dr. John Lee, author of *What Your Doctor May Not Tell You About Breast Cancer*: "When a cancer is first detectable by mammogram, it takes only a year or two for it to increase in size to be detectable by palpation (hand). This two-year time interval, statistics have shown, has little effect on the likelihood of a breast cancer to metastasize (spread through the lymph or blood system to other parts of the body). This is why routine mammography for low-risk patients has little effect on ultimate mortality from breast cancer. Recent studies have clearly shown that mammography is of dubious value, and that women can probably achieve the same benefit by carefully examining their own breasts each month."

A woman with an aggressive form of cancer would cringe about Dr. Lee's view on timing of detection, but most cancer is slow-growing. However, with the Plexus Breast Chek Kit, that time interval may be much less, as it often finds lumps earlier than even mammography. And as you will learn in secret 14, there is something you can do to detect breast problems 8 to 10 years before mammography is able to.

So the whole issue of taking breast health back into your own hands involves more than checking your breasts for cancer every month.

It means becoming educated about your breasts and hormonal system. Many women understand the workings of their cell phone or computer better than their own body. Consequently, they accept being placated by a medical system that insists that interfering with this very delicate balance poses no harm or risk. An educated woman asks more questions, does not accept blanket statements without proof, and questions the tests, the procedures and the protocols recommended, until *she* feels satisfied with the decisions she ultimately makes.

Reading this book is one part. Becoming part of the Breast Health Revolution is another, where there is a plethora of resources and education on breast health. Ignorance is no excuse, and far too many women start learning about their breasts after they hear the word cancer. Wouldn't it be far better to learn how to care for this most precious part of your body now, so you never have to hear those words? That is my desire for every woman on the planet and I know that *together* we can make it reality. Doing a monthly BSE is one way that you can begin to take breast health back into your own hands, but do it with knowledge, empowerment and a knowingness that your body has a remarkable ability to heal itself.

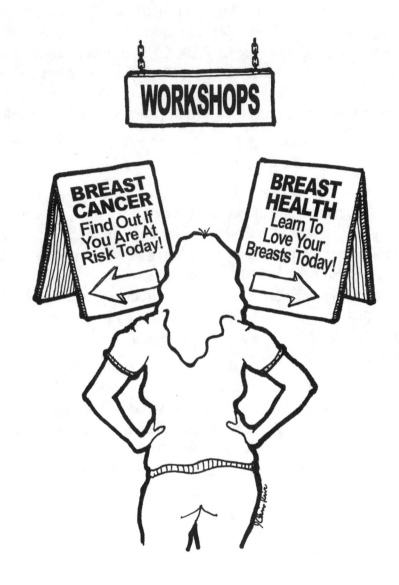

Breast Health Exposed

Secret #10:

Get Alkaline

Our bodies have a very important and delicate pH balance that needs to be maintained to achieve optimum health. Unfortunately the typical diet today is comprised mostly of acidic foods, which is playing havoc with our health. Cancer cells thrive in an acidic environment and cannot survive in an alkaline one, so this is something every woman wants to consider as part of her healthy breast program.

According to Dr. Robert Young, "A chronically over-acidic body pH corrodes body tissue, slowly eating into the 60,000 miles of our veins and arteries like acid eating into marble. If left unchecked, it will interrupt all cellular activities and functions, from the beating of your heart to the neural firing of your brain. Over-acidification interferes with life itself, leading to all sickness and disease."

Your body strives for a constant pH balance of 7.4 in the blood. It does this by automatically depositing and withdrawing acid and alkaline minerals from your bones, soft tissues, body fluids and saliva. When you eat more acidic food, your body need to take those alkaline minerals from your reserves, leaving you depleted of calcium, magnesium and potassium.

If you are consuming more acidic food than alkaline food, your body becomes overloaded with the burden of removing the acidic waste as your body works hard to maintain that perfect balance. That causes cells to be deprived of the nutrients they need and they either die or they adapt to the acidic environment and become abnormal, mutated cells that multiply indefinitely and without order. We call this cancer.

> ***There are simple ways to get the body back into that perfectly balanced state which leans slightly towards being more alkaline.***
>
> 1. Drink alkaline water. This means no tap water, and even some bottled water will be acidic.
>
> 2. Exercise. I love my rebounder and see my cells dancing with joy every time I bounce on it. More oxygen in my cells means cancer cannot thrive.
>
> 3. Fruits and vegetables are alkaline, as well as grains, nuts and seeds.

How do you create an alkaline environment in your body? One way is to remove some of the big culprits that are making you acidic. For example, a soda pop has a pH around 2, thus it is 100,000 (105) times more acidic than water with a pH of around 7. People who consume huge amounts of sodas (as well as coffee and alcohol) are typically very acidic.

It takes 32 glasses of alkaline water at an alkaline pH of 9 to neutralize the acid from just one 12-oz. cola or soda. When you drink a cola or soda, the body will use up reserves of its own stored alkaline buffers, mainly calcium from the bones and DNA to raise the body's alkalinity levels, especially to maintain proper blood alkaline pH levels.

If you are drinking soda pop, then just be aware of what it is doing to your pH levels. Also, the natural killer cells in your immune system will shut down for six hours after you consume just one teaspoon of sugar. There are 9 teaspoons of sugar in a 12-oz. soda pop! Needless to say, it takes a lot of work to bring your body back to normal. Is that soda pop worth it? Diet sodas are even worse because of the artificial sweeteners, so that is not the answer. Find alternatives such as water and lemon or lime or herbal teas. I love licorice herbal tea. Great for the adrenal glands (which helps deal with stress) and it tastes delicious.

Diet plays a huge part in your acid/alkaline levels. The typical developed country diet of processed foods, sugar (the average American right now eats ½ pound of sugar a day!), artificial sweeteners, alcohol, regular table salt, dairy and meat, including shellfish, all shift us towards the acidic side of the scale. Antibiotics are also very acidic, so be aware that you will be heading towards acidic if you take antibiotics before you even start eating and drinking. You will have extra acidity to compensate for to bring your body back to alkaline.

Fresh fruit, vegetables, whole grains, nuts and seeds bring you back to the alkaline side, so it's important to incorporate them into your diet.

It's easy to find out whether or not you are acidic or alkaline with a pH strip you can pick up at a pharmacy. Either used with saliva or urine, you can see exactly where you are at on the scale and watch how diet adjustments affect your acid/alkaline levels.

The aim is to ensure the pH level of your body is very slightly alkaline. Your body is at its healthiest at a pH of about 7.2 - 7.4.

Remember: Everyone with cancer has acidic (low) blood pH levels.

Another very easy thing can help. Although it would seem exactly the contrary, vinegar and lemons actually alkalize our bodies.

Having a teaspoon of raw organic, unrefined apple cider vinegar three times a day will be of benefit. You can put it into a glass of water and it is very palatable. I make myself a cup of hot water in the morning with some lemon or lime. You could also add a slice of ginger if you like. This is one of my most favorite drinks.

The subject of alkalinity has become a very hot and controversial health topic. We've seen a tremendous amount of education geared to helping us get alkaline and stay youthful, despite the aging process. Although you can read entire books on this subject, by putting the very simple tips in this chapter into practice, you will be well on your way to an ideal pH level. That means oxygenated cells which send out a very clear message to cancer: You are not welcome here! But there very well could be other side benefits to your breast health, simply by getting alkaline. Fibrocystic breast condition or other cyst conditions in the breasts can vanish by just applying this one secret!

You're doing great by getting this far. Your breasts are worth it, aren't they?

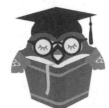

8 Ways to Stay Alkaline
from
Dr. Richard A. DiCensco

1. Drink plenty of water.

2. Eat lots of vegetables.

3. Avoid deep fried foods.

4. Avoid refined sugar.

5. Avoid refined carbs (white bread, white pasta, white rice).

6. Avoid chemical additives in food.

7. Eat slowly, chew thoroughly.

8. Never skip meals.

Secret #11:

Watch What You Put On Your Body

A s we slather lotions on our skin, bathe in magical potions, decorate our nails and beautify our face with jars of proven science, it's hard to believe that we are actually poisoning ourselves. I mean, isn't it all tested, proven and backed up with expensive scientific studies? The reality is a far cry from what most women think.

Let's start with two critically important points

1. Everything you put on your body gets absorbed through the skin and your body then needs to deal with the chemicals, toxins and veritable cornucopia of substances that can make up one simple body lotion or shampoo.

2. Just because it hasn't been declared Dangerous, Poisonous or doesn't bear a Warning label, doesn't mean it's safe.

When the U.S. Congress ordered the banning of PCB's in 1976, it also passed the Toxic Substances Control Act, (TSCA), which authorized the U.S. Environmental Protection Agency to approve and regulate new chemicals. Approximately 58,000 existing chemicals were grand-fathered in, no questions asked, including PBDE's. (Polybrominated diphenyl ethers are organobromine compounds that are used as flame retardants and are classified as potential human carcinogens.)

The trade publication for environmental, health and safety works, *EHS Today*, reports that the TSCA's greatest weakness is its inability to stop dangerous chemicals from entering the market. "Under current policy, the [Environmental Protection Agency] can call for safety testing only after evidence surfaces demonstrating a chemical is dangerous. As a result, EPA has been able to require testing for just 200 of the more than 80,000 chemicals currently registered in the United States and has been able to ban only five dangerous substances."

Right now there are about 2,000 new chemicals proposed every year and limited data to review. The federal agency is seriously behind in their testing. Interestingly, Europe is way ahead of North America, as they use something called the Precautionary Principle. In other words, manufacturers have to prove something is safe before it can be approved. In the U.S., the exact opposite is true. It's approved and then everybody hopes for the best!

So the assumption that if it is in a product, it must be safe, is simply not true and leads women into a false sense of security around the products she is buying for her family, her house and her daily personal care products.

According to Dr. Sherrill Sellman, author of *What Women MUST Know to Protect Their Daughters From Breast Cancer*, the word non-toxic appears on many consumer products but this is misleading. Non-toxic doesn't mean – "not at all toxic" or "absolutely safe." It means that up to half (as opposed to more than half) of the laboratory animals exposed to the product through ingestion or inhalation died within two weeks. A product can also be called non-toxic if no serious (immediate) damage occurred through eye or skin contact. These tests reflect only short-term health effects that may be associated with the product. Long-term or chronic effects are not considered.

In Canada, there are no regulations as to what non-toxic means. They leave it up to the consumer to decide. Nice, hey?

What does this mean for you and your breasts? First of all, think pure (not natural or even organic) as there are sketchy regulations there, also. Secondly, understand that it is the "wild west" when it comes to product evaluation and safety.

According to the Environmental Working Group (EWG), in just the first hour of the day, the average adult uses nine products and is subjected to 126 chemicals.

Think through your day and notice how many chemicals you are putting on your body.

- Shampoo and conditioner
- Mousse or gel
- Soap
- Toothpaste
- Mouthwash
- Moisturizer
- Deodorant
- Perfume
- Make-up

According to the EWG, only about 11 percent of the approximately 10,500 chemical ingredients used in the personal care products we assume are safe have actually been tested for safety. And it's the remaining 89 percent of untested ingredients which are used in more than 99 percent of all products on the market.

Start by replacing some of your products with purer products. One easy place to start is to remove all anti-bacterial soaps from your house. The chemical triclosan that is in thousands of household and personal care products has been linked to endocrine disrupting properties. In other words, it messes with your hormones! Now labeled a potential carcinogen and banned in Europe, the FDA has spent over 30 years examining the studies and says it is still three years away from publishing any conclusion. In the meantime, this chemical has been directly linked to the growth of human breast cancer cells. I highly suggest you not wait until the FDA makes up its mind but simply remove products with triclosan from your home.

Di-n-butyl phthalate (DBP): is used in cosmetics, hair sprays, nail polish and insect repellent. An environmental release of just 10 pounds of this toxic chemical must be reported to environmental authorities, yet thousands of tons of it is used in nail polish every year and no reporting is required.

Small changes such as not wearing toxic perfume or switching to safe nail polishes, purer shampoos and toothpastes can lessen the load. Eliminate those air fresheners in your house and open the window instead. You really need to get rid of the notion that you need chemically laden products to smell "nice" in your genitals, underarms, and mouth; your clothes and house. The truth is that you are paying a very high price with your health and the health of your children for that "nice, clean, fresh scent" you have been programmed to believe you need.

Instead I strongly urge starting with a bottle of vinegar and some good old 3% hydrogen peroxide and using that for most cleaning projects, including your house, clothes and body. We have this notion that we can't afford to "go organic" – but if you added up the price of all those products, vinegar, water and some hydrogen peroxide are pennies on the dollar. More importantly, your body doesn't have to deal with all the chemicals you are pouring into them, slathering on them and subjecting them to daily.

A good thing to remember is that everything is absorbed through the skin and filtered through the liver, so the more toxic the products you are using, the more strain on your immune system. A strong and healthy immune system is what keeps you and your breasts happy and healthy, so take care of it by lessening the load it must carry. Just breathing and living today is hard work for your immune systems.

Secret #12:

Love Your Breasts

What do you think about your breasts? If you had to describe your breasts, what would you say? Would you describe them as perky, beautiful, voluptuous, sexy, gorgeous or fabulous? At the other end of the spectrum, would you say they were ugly, lopsided, too big, too small or awkward?

Unfortunately due to an abundance of media around breasts, women have this idea of what the "perfect" breast should look like. However, while recently researching on a website, I saw that the author had a photo gallery of women's breasts. The purpose? To show women the wide range of perfectly normal breasts. Breasts are as individual as we are.

It's hard to believe that you may be the only woman who doesn't have a model's breasts or the most photogenic breasts in the world. But that is simply not true. Breasts come in all shapes and sizes.

In working with hundreds of women who experienced either inappropriate sexual behavior or sexual abuse in childhood or in their teen years, I have noted in my own private practice that many women hold negative emotions within the reproductive organs of their body.

As a medical intuitive, I can "see" inside the body and sense various problems with organs. I have helped clients deal with many physical issues that include painful periods, constipation or painful intercourse. In working with women who have been sexually abused to some degree in their life, there is often an abhorrence or revulsion around their sexual organs, including the vagina, uterus and breasts, conscious or unconscious. Emotions of guilt, anger, fear and sadness are common.

I vividly recall one client who had just had a mastectomy, and she told me that her grandfather had fondled her breasts as a young girl. Her comment to me was, "I just wanted to cut them off." As she said that, she consciously had no connection with the fact that she had just accomplished her wish.

Two University of California researchers noted associations between early sexual abuse and several health conditions in the elderly. Murray B. Stein and co-author Elizabeth Barrett-Connor, MD, analyzed health data on more than 1,300 elderly white, middle-class study participants from a Southern California community. More than 12 percent of the women and 5 percent of the men reported early sexual abuse. Most of the respondents never received counseling for their experience. Past sexual assault was associated with an increased risk of breast cancer, arthritis and thyroid disease. The findings varied by gender. In women, early sexual assault appeared to increase the risk of arthritis and breast cancer, with multiple abuse episodes increasing disease risk by two- to three-fold compared with a single episode.

Another study of 94 women with metastatic or recurring breast cancer discovered that nearly 42% of them had what was considered a traumatic life event.

Do I believe that all breast issues are emotional? If it was only that easy. However, I do firmly believe, after working with over a thousand clients, that emotions are at the root of many physical issues.

Unresolved anger, unforgiveness, or suppression of your emotions contribute to physical unease, leading to disease. Results of one study, based on statistical comparisons between 69 patients found to have breast cancer and a control group comprising the remaining 91 patients with benign breast disease, showed a significant association between the diagnosis of breast cancer and a behavior pattern. The pattern? An abnormal release of emotions. This abnormality was, in most cases, extreme suppression of anger and, in patients over 40, extreme suppression of other feelings.

Dr. Ben Johnson, oncologist and author of *The Secret of Health – Breast Wisdom,* says he has never seen a cancer that didn't have an underlying issue of lack of forgiveness. Dr. Alex Lloyd, developer of *The Healing Codes*, says that virtually every type of sickness is rooted in an inability to forgive others or one's self for perceived wrongs.

Those are strong statements. Whether or not you agree with them, it will only benefit your overall health including your breast health if you show your breasts some love, perhaps forgiveness and tender loving care.

How can you do this?

1. Breasts like to be touched. If you never touch your breasts except to wash them, then begin by touching your breasts using a natural cream. I personally use Dr. Spencer's Breast Cream as it contains LOVE as the first ingredient, Bulgarian Rose Oil and Spirulina Algae. It feels wonderful and is specifically designed for breast use.

2. Talk to your breasts. Just like a child constantly reprimanded to feel useless and worthless often turns delinquent as a fulfillment of the constant message, your breasts need to feel loved and appreciated. I enjoy telling my breasts how beautiful they are, how much I love them and how appreciated they are right where they are.

3. Speak highly of yourself overall. If you are constantly saying negative things about yourself such as, "I am so stupid. I am constantly doing dumb things. I am useless or worthless," you are programming every cell of your body to fulfill that negative message. Replace your language with comments about your attributes, what you do well and build your self-esteem constantly. Associating with people who instill confidence and self-worth in you and your body image is important to this secret.

4. Look at yourself naked in the mirror and celebrate your beautiful, sexy, luscious or gorgeous breasts, whatever shape or size they are. And for those of you who have lost a breast or breasts to cancer, I still encourage you to massage your chest area, talk to your body and love yourself.

When was the last time you thought of your breasts with appreciation and admiration for being part of your body? Spend a couple of minutes and just think about how you feel about your breasts and make a commitment today to start really loving and appreciating your beautiful breasts.

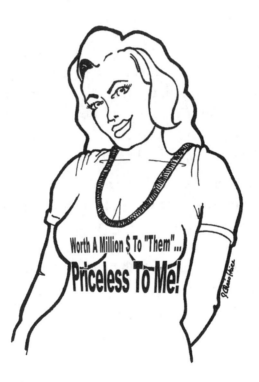

Secret #13:

Mammography Can Cause Breast Cancer

This secret may be one of the more controversial, as so many women are passionate about the importance of regular mammograms; and, certainly, the medical establishment, cancer organizations and charities endorse them heartily. So before you hang me by my toenails for this one, let me give you some information that seems to go "missing" when organizations or doctors have a vested interest in mammography.

Dr. Ben Johnson, oncologist, writes in his book: *The Secret of Health – Breast Wisdom*: "What your doctor won't tell you is that a mammogram exposes you to approximately 1,000 times the amount of radiation you'd get in a chest X-ray. If that's not enough, the radiation is stored in your cells and so it accumulates to significant levels over time, if you're getting an annual mammogram."

Sister Rosalie Bertell, one of the world's most respected authorities on the dangers of radiation, says one rad increases breast cancer risk one percent and is the equivalent of one year of natural aging.

The usual dose of radiation during a mammographic x-ray is from 0.25 to 1 rad with the very best equipment. That's 1 to 4 rads per screening mammogram (two views per breast). And according to Samuel Epstein, M.D. of the University of Chicago's School of Public Health, the dose can be ten times more than that.

Susun Weed, author of *Breast Cancer? Breast Health!*, says: "Scientists agree that there is no safe dose of radiation. Cellular DNA in the breast is more easily damaged by very small doses of radiation than thyroid tissue or bone marrow. Breast cells are second only to fetal tissues in sensitivity to radiation. And the younger the breast cells, the more easily their DNA is damaged by radiation. As an added risk, one percent of American women carry a hard-to-detect oncogene, which is triggered by radiation; a single mammogram increases their risk of breast cancer by a factor of 4-6 times."

In 1974, while mammography was in its infancy, the National Cancer Institute was warned by Professor Malcolm C. Pike at the University of Southern California School of Medicine that a number of specialists had concluded that "giving a women under age 50 a mammogram on a routine basis was close to unethical." This warning was ignored.

So how much radiation are we really talking about? For example:

One week at a high altitude (Denver) = less than 1 millirad

Jet flight of six hours = 5 millirads

Chest x-ray = 16 millirads (about 1 millirad reaches breast tissue)

Smallest possible dose from a screening mammogram done with the best possible equipment = 340 millirads

In the 2008/2009 annual report of the President's Cancer Panel released in May, 2010, they reported that "people who receive multiple scans or other tests that require radiation **may accumulate doses equal to or exceeding that of Hiroshima atomic bomb survivors**. It is believed that a single large dose of ionizing radiation and numerous low doses equal to the single large dose have much the same effect on the body over time." These scans and tests would include CT scans, x-rays and mammograms. (emphasis added by author)

If a woman has yearly mammograms from age 55 to age 75, she will receive a minimum of 20 rads of radiation. For comparison, women, who survived the atomic bomb blasts in Hiroshima or Nagasaki, absorbed 35 rads. By the way, damage from radiation is cumulative, so dental x-rays, CT scans, mammograms and any other exposure to radiation, including flying, all count.

Imagine the amount of radiation a woman would receive if she followed the current advice of many doctors and organizations that still suggests annual screening from the age of 40! Could this high level of radiation be one simple, preventable reason for the increase of breast cancer? However, there is another concern few take into consideration.

Dr. William Campbell Douglass Jr. reports: "Although the principle of handling cancer very gently so as not to spread it is widely accepted by the medical profession, it doesn't apply to breast screening. During mammography, the techniques used are designed for maximum detection of abnormalities without regard to the possible consequences of the action." Douglass notes a survey that found mammographers used as much compression as the patient could tolerate and had no idea how much compression they were using. In fact, the guidelines for mammography state that "adequacy of the compression device is crucial to good quality mammography." That force is 300 newtons, the equivalent of placing a 50 pound weight on the breast." Dr. Douglass reports one animal study that found that the number of metastases will increase by 80 percent if the tumor is manipulated. A human study reported in the *British Medical Journal* found that death rates were increased by 29 percent in women whose breasts were squeezed during mammography. This is likely to be the result of the rupture of small blood vessels in or around small, yet undetected, breast cancers. This squeezing into the blood stream of malignant cells is why many women with breast cancer have cancer cells in their lymph nodes.

So your squeamishness around the pain of having your breasts compressed in a mammogram is an honest concern. But isn't mammography the best tool for early detection?

No, mammography is in fact, LATE detection. By the time a cancer is big enough to be seen on a mammogram, it's usually eight years old, has 500 million cells, and is approximately one-quarter inch (half a centimeter) long. Breast cancers generally don't begin to metastasize until they contain at least 1 million cells. It takes an ordinary breast cancer—one that doubles every 100 days—about six years to grow that large. A million cells is only as big as the period at the end of a sentence and can't be detected by touch (without the Plexus Breast Chek Kit) or a mammogram. Mammography not only causes breast cancer but it doesn't even find it early!

You may be thinking that this is highly over-exaggerated, but I assure you the risks are real. Just ask Carol Conti. Carol was one of the first registered Mammographers in the United States. For over 10 years she has overseen the licensing of all Radiologic Technologists in the state of Arizona. So Carol knows a few things about mammography, having done them for 36 years! Carol also was diagnosed with breast cancer in the summer of 2009. Interestingly, the mammogram saw nothing. It was a thermogram that indicated there was a problem. So Carol returned for an ultrasound, which found the mass and discovered the fast-growing cancer. Carol blames the 30 mammograms for her breast cancer, as she knows first-hand that radiologists are told to minimize the risks and the dosages. But the truth is: Every mammogram increases your risk of breast cancer 1 to 3%. Here's further proof.

Breast cancer rates increased significantly in four Norwegian counties after women began getting mammograms every two years. In fact, the start of screening mammography programs throughout Europe has been associated with increased incidences of breast cancer.

Is it possible that the exposure to radiation through mammography is actually causing the increase in breast cancer? Mammography started in the 1970's with women being sold on the benefits and none of the risks. Is it simply coincidental that breast cancer has steadily increased over the last four decades, and it has nothing to do with the increase in radiation exposure due to mammography and a host of other common medical tests such as CT scans that now include radiation? I think not.

However, it doesn't mean you need to be left vulnerable. As a matter of fact, there is a much better way to detect breast cancer early. It's the next secret.

Secret #14:

Choose Thermography

If every woman could have a wish list when it came to her breast health, surely it would include knowing about any potential problems long before they became serious. It would include pain-free, risk-free detection, and the time, ability and knowledge to eliminate the problem under the guidance of a knowledgeable and supportive medical team.

You may be surprised that something, which fits the bill precisely, does exist and has for some time. It's called thermography. Dr. Len Saputo describes thermograpy in his report, "Beyond Mammography" this way: "Thermography measures differences in infrared heat emission from normal breast tissue, benign breast abnormalities—such as fibrocystic disease, cysts, infections and benign tumors—and from breast cancers. Modern infrared scanners (cameras) have a thermal sensitivity of 0.05 degrees Centigrade. When the breast is cooled with small fans in a room kept at 68 degrees Fahrenheit, blood vessels of normal tissue respond by constricting to conserve heat while tumor tissue remains hot. Thus, tumors emit more heat than their surrounding tissues and are usually easily detected by heat-sensing infrared scanners."

As cancer cells develop (before a mass or tumor forms), they release chemicals into the surrounding area to stimulate more blood flow. The cancer cells will build a network of blood flow to the areas it plans to call home.

These chemicals help to:

- Keep existing blood vessels wide open,
- Wake up "sleeping" blood vessels, and
- Create new blood vessel growth.

The increased blood flow will increase the heat in these areas. As thermography detects the hot spots in your breasts created by this blood flow, you and your doctor will receive the earliest clues possible as to what is happening in your breasts.

A mammogram can only tell you what is already present in your breast in the form of a lump. A clinical breast exam, or one you do on your own, can only find what has already created a tumor. Thermography is different because it can assess a woman's risk of developing a tumor up to 10 years BEFORE it actually happens. It is also the only non-invasive test that can assess your hormonal status.

Dr. Ben Johnson, author of *The Secret of Health – Breast Wisdom*, says about this important factor: "As one of the greatest risk factors for the development of breast cancer is total lifetime exposure to estrogen, normalizing the balance of the hormones in the breast may be the first and most significant step in prevention. Breast thermography is the only known non-invasive procedure that can detect estrogen dominance in the breasts."

Thermography detects temperature differences that can occur when cancers have grown to 200-300 cells in size, while mammography detects cancers only once they reach a size of 500 million cells. The difference between finding something 200-300 cells in size compared with 500,000,000 is huge!

Research has shown thermography to be 97% sensitive in finding abnormalities in breast tissue, including the earliest stages of breast cancer. In contrast, mammography is reported to miss 50% of tumors in dense breast tissue, 30% of tumors in fibrocystic breasts, and 10-15% of tumors in fatty (normal) breasts.

A thermogram is an early warning system that will let you know you are on the wrong road, if you want to have healthy breasts, 5, 10, 20 years down the path. As breast cancer can take 15 years to develop, this kind of lead-time to see potential problems could save many lives. Thermography gives you time to look at factors that may be contributing to the problems, such as hormonal challenges, a lifestyle or diet that needs some improving or a major tune-up of your critically important immune system.

Currently, there are thermographers in the U.S. who are having their patients use Dr. Spencer's Breast Cream, which has been effective in eliminating many of the potential problems in their breasts. After only 90 days of using the cream, subsequent thermograms are showing either remarkable improvement or a complete clearing of issues. Needless to say, this could be a huge bonus to women using Dr. Spencer's Breast Cream on a regular basis as part of their daily breast health program.

Unlike mammography, thermography can also distinguish between fibrocystic breasts and cancerous tumors. It can examine breasts with implants, which cannot be adequately screened with routine mammography because the compression could damage the implant and because the implant can actually block the view of deeper parts of the breast. It is effective for breasts of all sizes, whereas mammography can be inaccurate for women with very small or very large breasts. It's also not affected by denser breast tissues, which is a problem with mammography.

It is non-invasive, pain-free and there is no radiation, but has it been proven? If you listen to strong advocates of mammography, especially those with a vested interest in it, you would think thermography was the latest "kid on the block" with no proven track record. That's just not so.

More than 800 research papers have been published on the subject of breast thermography, and a research databank on more than 300,000 women, who have been tested with infrared breast imaging, now exists. The FDA has approved it as a breast cancer risk assessment tool since 1982. Mammography wasn't approved until 1989.

Women who have been given a clean bill of health with a mammogram have used thermography to verify their own intuition that the doctor's statement that "everything is fine" just wasn't true, or to clarify results that were ambiguous. This is precisely what happened with Carol Conti, mentioned in the last chapter. Although Carol's mammogram showed nothing abnormal and she was assured that her breasts were healthy, her own breast self-exam, confirmed by a thermogram, proved otherwise. Carol is now a leading thermographer in the state of Arizona and is working hard to "undo the damage" she feels she contributed to by advocating mammography for decades.

Thermography does an excellent job of providing an early, accurate picture of your breast, and women as young as 25 are encouraged to get their baseline thermogram and then monitor their breast health regularly. These images are unique to each woman and remain stable over time, which is why changes are much easier to see over a woman's lifetime. Men can have thermograms, too, and thermography is ideal for the entire body.

Are you convinced that thermography is a powerful tool for early detection of breast cancer and should be made available free of cost to every woman? So why isn't it?

Dr. Sherri Tenpenny says: "Thermography's only error is that it is 'too early.' The tools to address a positive thermogram include diet, exercise, iodine, and other nutraceuticals that conventional doctors know little, if anything, about. It is in this capacity that the paradigm must shift."

Does Dr. Tenpenny really mean thermography is too early? It's not too early for the woman who now has up to a decade of time to deal with the breast issues before they become a problem, who can have non-invasive, risk-free testing done and get an accurate picture of her breast health. To her, this is a dream come true!

Secret #15:

Check Your Iodine Level

Perhaps you have cut back on your salt intake over the last few years, in light of studies which show that too much salt is a bad thing.

While the highly processed salt we get in processed foods is definitely a culprit for a number of health factors, unfortunately when we threw out the salt, we also threw out the iodine.

Up until the 1980's, iodine was commonly used in bakery products. However, due to a concern that we were getting too much iodine, bromine replaced iodine in baked goods. Additionally mineral-deficient soils are now the norm, meaning that our vegetables don't have the minerals and vitamins, including iodine, necessary for optimal health.

According to many medical doctors and studies, this decrease in iodine very well could be a bottom line cause of many diseases including breast cancer, prostate cancer, and thyroid problems.

Every organ in your body needs iodine, with the thyroid taking whatever iodine there is to take first. However in an iodine-deficient state, the thyroid gland and the breasts will compete for whatever iodine is to be found, because after the thyroid, the highest concentration of iodine is found in a woman's breast tissue. Studies with animals have shown conclusively that an iodine-deficient state can alter the structure and function of the breasts.

Japan and Iceland have higher intakes of iodine and lower rates of goiter and breast cancer. Countries such as the U.S., Mexico and

Thailand have lower iodine intake and higher incidences of both breast cancer and goiter. There's something to the fact that parts of the world with the lowest iodine in their diets have been found to have very high rates of breast cancer.

So although Japan's low breast cancer rate is often attributed to their consumption of soy products, I propose that the lower rate of breast cancer has less to do with soy and more to do with iodine. In view of the actually very small amount of soy products that the Japanese eat and the high levels of sea vegetables they consume, it might be the more accurate conclusion, although certainly not the most profitable for big corporations that have a vested interest in soy.

Are we actually deficient in iodine? The RDA (Recommended Daily Allowance) for iodine is seriously low, according to Dr. David Brownstein, an expert in iodine. He's not the only doctor who feels that iodine deficiency is causing serious health problems and the dosage needs to be raised. Currently, the RDA is 150 mcg a day. Yet Dr. Guy Abraham, one of the world's leading researchers on iodine, states that we need 13 mg per day. The thyroid glands need approximately 6 mg/day; and remember, the thyroid picks first so if your thyroid is not getting sufficient iodine, your breasts aren't getting any!

The breasts need at least 5 mg of iodine, leaving 2 mg per day for the rest of your body.

Dr. Brownstein feels that every woman, and especially every woman with breast cancer, should have her iodine levels tested. Most doctors are simply not aware of the latest research on iodine because it isn't linked with a pharmaceutical company's newest drug. Consequently, you very well may be more informed than your medical doctor.

There's a whole other side to the iodine deficiency story. There are certain toxic substances that you are subjected to daily that deplete any of your iodine reserves. This means that even if you are getting a higher than average amount of iodine in your body, through excellent sources such as natural sea salt and seaweed for example, there are robbers that are stealing it right from under your nose.

Crazily enough, one is the very chemical the food industry chose to replace iodine with—bromine. Bromine is found in many food items such as bakery products and some sodas, as well as many prescription items. Bromine is in many fire-retardant chemicals, added to furniture, carpets, hot tubs and pools.

A small study, comparing the bromide levels of breast cancer patients with a control group without breast cancer, showed bromide levels were nearly two times higher in the breast cancer group. You can see why ensuring you have sufficient iodine is critically important.

Fluoride is another thief of iodine. Fluoride is known to be a toxic agent and has been shown to inhibit the ability of the thyroid gland to concentrate iodine. Many commonly prescribed medications contain fluoride including Paxil and Prozac and it's found in most municipality water supplies.

Low iodine, combined with high bromine and fluoride, is a perfect recipe for breast cancer. And today, that's a recipe most women are cooking!

Chlorine used in community water, swimming pools and hot tubs as a disinfectant also robs your body of iodine. You may know it most commonly as the whitener in bleach. A byproduct of chlorine is dioxin. Dioxin is one of the most toxic carcinogens known to mankind. Even the steam of the dishwasher when the door is opened after cleaning (chlorine superheated and combined with detergent) is toxic. Another common product on the market today, Splenda, also contains chlorinated table sugar and will deplete your body of vital iodine.

"We think it's very important for the breast," says Dr. Stephen A. Hoption Cann, PhD, University of British Columbia. This mineral, he believes, may prevent and even shrink breast tumors by combining with certain fatty acids and stopping cancerous cells from multiplying. You can see the power of this dynamic duo in Japan, where people eat about 5 grams of sea vegetables virtually every day. Cann points out that the Japanese have one of the highest life expectancies, as well as a very low rate of breast cancer.

It has also been found that iodine lowered several estrogen responsive genes. Iodine increased BRCA1 activity. BRCA1 is a gene that modulates estrogen activity in the breast. People with abnormalities in BRCA1 are at a markedly increased risk for breast cancer.

Dr. Bernard Eskin, PhD and expert in iodine and breast disease, has studied the effects of estrogen and iodine in rats. He has found that rats need an adequate level of iodine in order for estrogen to perform its normal function in breast tissue. Rats given certain carcinogens will develop breast cancer. When iodine is given along with the carcinogens, tumor formation is blocked.

The foods richest in iodine are dulse and kelp. All sea vegetables basically contain all of the minerals of the sea, bringing us a good source of trace minerals in general. Although you may not be ready to start eating seaweed, you can start by using sea salt (not the highly processed table salt) and supplementing with kelp capsules as readily accessible, economical ways to get more iodine in your body.

What is obvious from the research on iodine: It is impossible to have a balanced hormonal system without ensuring an adequate iodine intake.

Dr. Brownstein suggests that "Perhaps the reason we have made so little progress in our treatment of nearly all of the hormone-sensitive cancers is that the underlying cause has been overlooked. The underlying cause could very well be iodine deficiency."

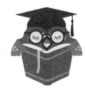

"Your breasts need at least 5 mg of iodine per day!"
–Dr. Guy Abraham

Secret #16:

Soy Is Not Good For Your Breasts

A costly media campaign led by massive soy producers has led most people to believe that soy is good for us and will decrease the risk of breast cancer. This actually couldn't be further from the truth.

Soybeans are not a complete protein, are not a natural food, contain several harmful and even carcinogenic substances, and most soybeans in the United States are genetically modified.

Dr. Jonathon Wright, a Harvard-trained medical doctor who is a pioneer in natural medicine is very blunt when he says: "Until the 1930's, the only place in the U.S. where you could find soybeans was at your local hardware store—in your paint and varnish." He continues, "Unlike other legumes, soybeans aren't safe to eat when picked fresh. They're actually toxic. In order to remove the harmful toxins, manufacturers must use harsh chemical processing. The beans are subject to acid baths and extreme heat, then they're spray dried to produce a high protein powder. Next, to improve the taste of the soy powder, artificial flavorings such as MSG, preservatives, sweeteners, emulsifiers and synthetic nutrients are added."

Doctor Wright confirms the effect of soy on women's delicate hormonal systems: "One hundred grams of soy protein daily—the amount recommended by a national soy organization—provides the estrogenic equivalent of taking the birth control pill."

Joseph Mercola, MD, warns: "Drinking even two glasses of soymilk daily for one month has enough phytoestrogens to alter a woman's menstrual cycle, and although the FDA regulates estrogen-containing products, no warnings exist on soy."

Today with most soy products being genetically modified, this leads to even more serious issues. When GMO (genetically modified) soy was fed to female rats, most of their babies died within three weeks— compared to a 10% death rate among the control group fed natural soy. The GMO-fed babies were also smaller, and later had problems getting pregnant. When male rats were fed GMO soy, their testicles actually changed color—from the normal pink to dark blue. Mice fed GMO soy had altered young sperm. Even the embryos of GMO-fed parent mice had significant changes in their DNA. By the third generation, the latest studies are showing the massive problem of sterility when rats are fed GMO food, including soy.

Now, I know we're not rats, but these findings are significant because GMO foods have not been fully tested. You are the guinea pig, and these findings are alarming, due to the important role hormones play in your breast health. Women need to understand breast health begins in the womb. With a male baby, the hormonal effects of the soy may be readily apparent in malformed genitalia. However, with girls, it may not show up for years or even decades later.

What alarmed me the most in the world of soy is the number of women feeding their infants soy formula, believing they are giving them the better alternative. However, "the amount of phytoestrogens that are in a day's worth of soy infant formula equals 5 birth control pills," says Mary G. Enig, Ph.D., president of the Maryland Nutritionists Association. She and other nutrition experts believe infant exposure to high amounts of phytoestrogens is associated with early puberty in girls and retarded physical maturation in boys.

Although in North America, soy is still hailed as a natural wonder, that is not the case everywhere.

"The Israelis have taken the strongest and most courageous stance of any government to date, warning that infants should not receive soy formula, that children up to age 18 should not eat soy foods or drink soy milk more than once per day to a maximum of 3 times per week and that adults should exercise caution because of adverse effects on fertility and increased breast cancer risk."

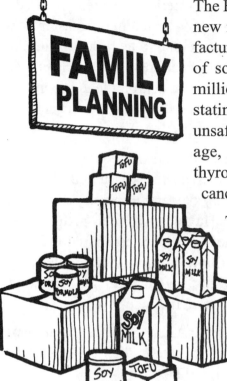

The French government is implementing new regulations that will require manufacturers to reduce the isoflavone content of soy infant formula to one part per million and will require warning labels stating that soy foods and soy milk are unsafe for children under three years of age, children being treated for hypothyroidism and women at risk for breast cancer.

The British Department of Health issued a warning back in 1996 that the phytoestrogens in soy-based infant formulas could adversely affect infant health. New Zealand has also taken a strong position against soy infant formulas. What are they privy to that other countries just aren't paying attention to?

Animal studies indicate health effects of possible concern include early onset of puberty in females and alterations in development of breast tissue. This statement comes from an American governmental agency— the National Institute of Environmental Health Sciences.

Elaine Hollingsworth, author of the best-seller *Take Control of Your Health and Escape the Sickness Industry,* is on the media constantly about the ill effects of soy. She reports, "I hear, almost daily, from parents whose baby daughters have commenced menstruation, developed pubic hair, underarm odor and breasts from as young as four and five years of age. Or whose teenage sons are too embarrassed to shower with their mates because they have grown breasts of female proportions or because their genitalia haven't developed." And if that isn't enough, she continues:

"The soy bean contains high levels of aluminum absorbed from the soil in which it is grown. In 1997, the American Academy of Pediatrics' Committee on Nutrition reported, "Aluminum in breast milk is 4 to 65 ng/mL. Soy-based formulas contain 600 to 1300 ng/mL," of this exceedingly dangerous mineral. As we discussed in the chapter on antiperspirants, aluminum has been linked to neurological, respiratory and reproductive diseases. Newborn babies should not be subjected to high amounts of aluminum in soy formulas, but they are.

So is all soy bad? As it is often reported that Asian people eat soy and they have less breast cancer than Americans, it is assumed people in Japan and China eat soy burgers every day and drink soy smoothies for breakfast. That is simply not true. Having traveled to both of these countries, their intake of soy products is minute compared to North Americans, and what they do consume is mostly fermented soy. Products such as miso, natto, tempeh and soy sauce are fermented soy and do not contain the health risks of unfermented soy.

However, a closer look at the truth of the Asian diet will reveal many characteristics, other than soy, that contribute to their lower rates of breast cancer, including a diet high in iodine.

We have been bamboozled by the media, regarding soy. Any study that says soy is safe has been funded or is in some way influenced by a major producer of soy. Genetically modified soy is of huge concern and, honestly, organic soy is dubious as well because of the prevalence of GMO soy and the wind spreading seed, even onto organic farms.

The truth is: Soy is not good for your breast health.

Secret #17:

Get Rid of the Candida

Do you crave sugar from the moment you get up in the morning? Does a piece of bread or a bowl of pasta make you think you've died and gone straight to heaven?

You may have candida. We all have this fungus/yeast in our bodies, but for many women (and men and kids), it is completely out of control and is causing havoc in your body.

An overgrowth of candida can cause vaginitis, migraines, asthma, fibromyalgia and cancer to name just a few of the problems!

When under control, it's harmless. The problem is that if your system is out of balance because your diet has been leaning heavily towards sugars and carbs, you've been on prescription drugs, or have been under excessive stress, candida is like a monster that can overtake you, and even kill. Seriously, if candida enters your bloodstream, it can be life threatening.

If candida overwhelms the good bacteria in your digestive tract, it can actually burrow into your intestinal wall. This creates tiny holes in the membrane lining. This is where it gets serious. There are 180 toxic byproducts of this fungus, all of which can escape the digestive tract and enter your bloodstream. Once in the bloodstream, the toxins are now delivered to every part of your body. Partially digested food particles go along for the ride and create leaky gut syndrome, which opens the door to a host of other diseases including depression, thyroid issues, autoimmune diseases, and weight gain.

What causes candida?

- Eating too much sugar and too many grains. Sugar feeds the fungus.

- Taking antibiotics, which kill both your good and bad bacteria.

- Exposure to environmental toxins, which lowers your immune system.

- Taking other medications, such as birth control pills.

- Chronic stress, diabetes and pregnancy, all of which impact your immune system and feeds the fungus.

It would be hard for anyone to not have made themselves susceptible to candida over the last 10 years, wouldn't you agree?

At some of her women's health workshops, nutritionist Brenda Eastwood takes a package of yeast used to make bread, puts it in water and then adds a teaspoon of sugar. The result is a smelly, foaming mess that inevitably overflows the cup. Many women may relate to this as looking very similar to a vaginal yeast infection. However, candida shows up in many ways.

Nipple issues while breast-feeding can also be a result of candida. You want to suspect candida if:

- Your nipples are extremely sore, burning, itching, red, or blistery.

- You experience shooting pains in your breasts during or just after feeding (especially during your milk ejection reflex).

- The usual remedies for sore nipples aren't working.

- Baby has oral thrush (white, cottage-cheese-like patches on the tongue and sides of the mouth) and/or a yeasty diaper rash.

- Your nipples suddenly become sore after a period of pain-free breastfeeding.

- You are taking, or have just finished taking, a course of antibiotics. Yeast infections are common following antibiotic treatment.

Adults can also get thrush, so if there are white, velvety sores in your mouth, that could be candida. Chemotherapy, which weakens the immune system, is one way you become susceptible to thrush.

But exactly how does candida affect your breast health? The more your body becomes overrun with candida, the more strain on your immune system. It becomes a losing battle as the enemy takes over. And once the candida enters the bloodstream, every organ is affected.

One Italian oncologist has made some fans for himself, and there are others who think he should be locked away. However, Dr. Simoncini's research has led him to believe that candida is the leading cause of cancer. This maverick doctor says that cancer itself is in fact a fungus, which, once it roots itself into your organs, creates a battle that your body eventually can't fight, and you die of cancer.

True or not, several studies have linked the presence of candida with cancer, showing that anywhere between 79 to 97 percent of all cancer patients also have candida. Candida and other fungus also excrete toxins that further weaken and damage the body.

The major waste product of candida is acetaldehyde, which produces ethanol. Now you'll see ethanol at the gas pump when you fill up your car. Needless to say, it should NOT be in your body! It causes excessive fatigue, destroys enzymes needed for cell energy, causes the release of free radicals that can damage DNA, and inhibits the absorption of iron.

Iron is critical to maintaining a healthy level of oxygen in your body. However, ethanol creates low oxygen levels in your body, and you've already learned that low oxygen is precisely where cancer comes to roost! A body full of candida is a perfect home for cancer. So do you have candida?

There is a simple test to tell if you have candida overgrowth.

First thing in the morning, before you put ANYTHING in your mouth, get a clear glass of water or leave it by your bed the night before. As soon as you wake up, work up a bit of saliva, and then spit it into the glass of water.

Check the water every <u>15 minutes</u> or so for up to one hour. If you have a candida yeast infection, strings (like legs) will travel down into the water from the saliva floating on top, or "cloudy" saliva will sink to the bottom of the glass, or cloudy specks will seem to be suspended in the water. If nothing develops in 30 to 45 minutes, you are probably candida free.

So how do you deal with candida? Three components are critical. A comprehensive combination of probiotics, (you need more than acidophilus and lactobacillus) enzymes to penetrate the fungus cell walls and natural anti-fungals such as grapefruit seed extract, oregano or garlic, which will kill the candida. Candida cleanses can be arduous, especially because a very strict diet usually accompanies the program. It's why I like the Plexus Pro-Bio 5. It's easier than anything else I've seen, effective, and very affordable. As this one can be overwhelming, time-consuming and costly, I wanted to support you by letting you know exactly what product I recommend in this case, because it is so important. I've actually spoken with the scientist who developed this product, and she is a brilliant woman with an impressive track record of success. It contains exactly what is needed to kill candida effectively.

If you have candida, you are strongly encouraged to eliminate the yeast and mold-containing foods from your diet. These include things such as alcohol, vinegar and anything that contains vinegar, such as mustard; also bread, carrots, potatoes and beets, as they all contain sugar; fruit, peanuts and corn, as they often contain mold; mushrooms, which are a fungus; and, aged cheeses. There is a diet recommended for candida at www.breasthealthrevolution.com/resources/nutrition.

There are several doctors, other than Dr. Simoncini, who believe that cancer is directly related to fungus. Candida is far more prevalent and serious than most family doctors will tell you. It may be a job you don't relish to bring your body into balance and eliminate the overgrowth of candida, but it is one that will affect not only your breast health, but EVERY area of your life. It may even save your life.

Secret #18:

Men Can Get Breast Cancer Too

Did you know that men can get breast cancer too? Although considered "rare" for men, breast cancer in men is increasing. Because of the overwhelming lack of awareness that even men can get breast cancer, the prognosis is often poor.

"Even though we don't think of men as having breasts, they have breast tissue and are susceptible to getting breast cancer," said Dr. Sharon Giordano, an associate professor of medicine in the department of breast medical oncology at the University of Texas M.D. Anderson Cancer Center in Houston.

"All men have some residual degree of breast tissue behind the nipples. It may be very small, but just like any part of the body can get cancer, that part of the body can get cancer," explains Dr. Giordano.

When compared to women, researchers found that men with breast cancer were on average 67 years of age versus 62 years for women. However, a young boy of seven, another of nine, had breast cancer, and men in their 30's and 40's have been diagnosed with it, so awareness cannot start too early.

It may be easier to find breast cancer in a male, but delays in the diagnosis can be deadly. Consequently, the disease is often discovered at an advanced stage, when the cancer has progressed to the lymph nodes. This results in a more serious prognosis.

So what do men need to look for? (This applies to women too, who are watching out for their men and sons.)

- a lump felt in the breast
- nipple pain
- an inverted nipple
- nipple discharge (clear or bloody) – more common in men with breast cancer than in women with the disease
- sores on the nipple and areola (the small ring of color around the center of the nipple)
- enlarged lymph nodes under the arm

Here are some factors that can increase a man's risk of getting breast cancer:

Age: Risk increases as age increases.

High estrogen levels, which can come from:

- Being overweight, which increases the production of estrogen.
- Estrogen in the environment (hormones in beef, dairy, the pesticide DDT, which can mimic the effects of estrogen in the body).
- Alcohol use. This is also true of women. However, one theory is that it could be the reduction of magnesium from alcohol use that increases the rate of cancer, rather than the alcohol itself. Low magnesium is a contributing factor to breast cancer.
- Liver disease. This usually leads to lower levels of androgens (male hormones) and higher levels of estrogen (female hormones).

Klinefelter syndrome: Normally men have a single X and a single Y chromosome. Men with Klinefelter syndrome have more than one X chromosome (sometimes as many as four). Symptoms include smaller than normal testicles, being infertile, a higher voice and a thinner beard. Again men with Klinefelter have a lower level of androgens and more estrogen. This puts them at a higher risk for breast cancer.

A strong family history of breast cancer: Family history can increase the risk of breast cancer in men—particularly if other men in the family have had breast cancer. Several researchers have reported two or more cases of male breast cancer within a single family. Several of these reports have involved two brothers; one involved three brothers; and another in a man, his father and his uncle.

Genetic Issues: The risk is also higher if there is a proven breast cancer gene abnormality in the family, such as men who inherit the BRCA1 or BRCA2 gene. However, the majority of male breast cancers happen in men who have no family history of breast cancer and no inherited gene abnormality.

Radiation exposure: If you had radiation therapy to the chest before 30, particularly during adolescence, or were treated with radiation for Hodgkin's disease, you may be at a higher risk of developing breast cancer. Ironically, the source where I found this information stated that radiation to treat breast cancer didn't count. However, radiation is radiation, and whether you get it from a dentist's visit, an airplane flight or a machine at a hospital, radiation is cumulative and dangerous. All radiation counts, even when it's used to treat breast cancer.

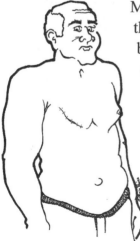

Most male breast cancers are not large. Perhaps this is another reason they get ignored. However, by using the Plexus Breast Chek Kit, which will detect a lump the size of a grain of salt, and by having thermograms, male breast cancer could be detected much earlier.

Some men have an enlargement of both their breasts. This is usually NOT cancer. The medical term for this is gynecomastia. Sometimes the breasts can become quite large and it can be embarrassing for men. Non-cancer-related enlargement of the breasts can be caused by medications, heavy alcohol use, weight gain, or marijuana use. However, there could be another reason not usually discussed.

Elaine Hollingsworth, an 83-year-old Australian actress, turned activist, is concerned about the misinformation around soy. One story she tells in her book, *Take Control of Your Health and Escape the Sickness Industry* is alarming. She writes, "A shocked mother described her son's tragic childhood. She had drunk copious amounts of soy milk during pregnancy—unknowingly poisoning her son with a female hormone. Then, because the estrogen had damaged her reproductive system, she was unable to breastfeed, and her baby received more from the soy baby formula her doctor told her to use. Her son's genitalia did not develop, but his breasts did and he refused to go to school until he had a double mastectomy. Unaware of the cause of their health problems, the family continued drinking soy milk and now, at 21, her son needs another double mastectomy, but they can't afford it."

My chapter on soy outlines serious implications for the hormonal balance in men, women and children. However, men, if you have growing breasts and are consuming soy products, you may want to look at this relatively unknown link.

For every person today, breast health is paramount. We all need to let the men we love know that they, too, need to take care of their breasts!

*We love
men's breasts
too!*

Secret #19:

Your Weight is Putting Your Breasts at Risk

With over two-thirds of the adults in the United States overweight or obese, a billion people overweight globally, and children becoming the fastest-growing obesity statistic, the weight loss industry is booming. Financially, it is predicted to be worth well over $500 billion U.S. dollars by 2014.

So what does obesity have to do with breast health? One of the risks for being overweight or obese is breast cancer.

According to Dr. Ben Johnson, author of *The Secret of Health - Breast Wisdom*, "Almost half of all breast cancer occurs in obese women. Overweight women are more likely to develop breast cancer because their bodies produce more estrogen than thin women do."

Before menopause, your ovaries produce most of your estrogen. Fat tissue also produces a small amount. Once you hit menopause and the ovaries no longer make estrogen, most of your estrogen will come from fat tissue. Logically, when there is more fat, there's more estrogen. Quite frankly, breast cancer wouldn't even be a topic of conversation without estrogen.

An aggressive type of breast cancer, known as inflammatory breast cancer, was also seen in significantly more obese and overweight patients than in normal-weight patients, according to a study, published in Clinical Cancer Research.

"The more obese a patient is, the more aggressive the disease," said principal investigator Dr. Massimo Cristofanilli of the University of Texas M.D. Anderson Cancer Center in Houston.

And what about mortality rates? After five years, the researchers report that 58.6 percent of the obese women, 58.3 percent of the overweight women and 69.3 percent of the normal-weight women were still alive.

After 10 years, 57.3 percent of the normal-weight or underweight had survived, compared with 42.4 percent of obese women and 44.1 percent of overweight women. So overweight women had a significantly lower survival rate than women who were a normal weight.

Another factor related to the higher breast cancer death rates in obese women is that breast cancer is more likely to be detected at a later stage in obese women than it is in thin women, because the detection of a breast tumor is simply more difficult.

Over 30 years ago, 120,000 female registered nurses, between the ages of 30 and 55, became involved in a study that has been going on for decades. The newest data obtained shows that weight loss after menopause does decrease the risk of breast cancer. The study included almost 50,000 of these women who noted their weight changes since menopause. Women who gained 55 pounds or more after age 18 had a 150% greater risk to get breast cancer, compared to woman who did not gain weight following their late teens. The women who stayed at the same weight from age 18 and then gained 22 pounds or more *after* menopause had an *18 percent increased risk of breast cancer, compared to the women who never gained weight.*

But the good news is that those women, who lost 22 pounds or more after menopause, had a 57 percent lower risk of breast cancer than the women who maintained their heavier weight. I don't know many women who haven't had their weight fluctuate since being a teen–but it is very encouraging that the risks can definitely be mitigated by losing the weight—at any age!

With breast cancer on the rise in both men and women, many factors have been considered in cancer detection—from the environment to the increased use of mammography. However, the increase in breast cancer has run parallel to the increase in obesity. Consequently, researchers surmise that between 11,000 and 18,000 breast cancer deaths per year could be avoided in American women over age 50, if they could maintain a healthy body weight throughout their adult lives.

With diabetes also on the increase, recent research shows that elevated insulin levels are an additional risk factor for breast cancer recurrence. High insulin levels are a contributing factor to weight gain, and excess weight will put you at a higher risk of breast cancer. However, women are not the only ones at risk. The newest concern is childhood obesity. Studies at various children's hospitals have shown that the earlier a girl begins breast development and menstruation, the higher her risk of breast cancer. What triggers early development? Being overweight in pre-puberty is one factor triggering the early onset of puberty in girls.

Overweight children generate early hormonal development, which increases the lifetime exposure to estrogen, which in turn increases breast cancer risk. Chubby kids are not cute. They are at a serious health risk and there will be a price to pay.

Paying a frighteningly high price, in 2009, a 10-year-old girl from California was diagnosed with breast cancer. She had a mastectomy and lymph nodes removed. Interestingly, in an interview her mother said, "Hannah had been wearing a bra for two years because of her larger size, although she was still pre-pubescent."

This may be a trend that becomes even more alarming as more and more young girls are affected by early puberty, an unhealthy diet and being overweight.

So, are diet pills, diet shakes, and drugs the answer? Noting that this is a half-trillion-dollar industry, it would be fairly easy to conclude that the vast majority of what people are doing isn't working. Diet pills can contain harmful chemicals and have side effects. Diet shakes are often full of chemicals. For example, artificial strawberry flavor can include as many as 40 different chemicals, and drugs inevitably go hand-in-hand with side effects. You can simply watch television in the U.S. to get a run-down on the long list of potential side effects with every drug recommended!

A diet full of fruit, vegetables, protein, healthy fats (such as coconut oil, olive oil), and complex carbohydrates (such as lentils and beans), would be the ideal diet. Many say that the Mediterranean diet is about as close to perfection as we will get. Obviously, exercise would also be part of the ideal combo. However, many need more help than that as they make adjustments to healthier eating.

So in looking for a weight loss product, look for something that does not contain caffeine or stimulants such as ephedra. If it's artificially flavored or contains aspartame, splenda or other artificial sweeteners, run in the other direction. Look for natural sweeteners such as stevia or lo han, a safe Chinese plant extract.

It also needs to be simple, as some weight loss programs have you mixing shakes and popping pills several times a day, or analyzing every mouthful of food with scientific scrutiny. It's easy to fall off the wagon when it's expensive, too complicated or overwhelming. Look for 'easy and simple' so you actually do it!

Is it worth the effort to lose those extra pounds? Right now, the U.S. is looking at a 334-billion-dollar bill by 2018, just for health issues related to obesity. No country in the world today can afford those kinds of repercussions from a society that has just grown bigger and bigger. Kids who are obese are at huge risk for type 2 diabetes, heart disease, renal failure and cancer, by their 30's. Old-people diseases will become commonplace for this generation of young people. Breast cancer will become a teenager's nightmare and girls will be going from training pants to sanitary napkins, with puberty starting as early as the age of seven.

It is imperative that we all bring our weight and fat ratios into a healthy range. We may not be able to change what chemicals are spewing into the environment today, but we are daily choosing what foods we are putting into our bodies. We need to choose wisely for our children and ourselves. Our breasts will be much happier as a result!

Secret #20:

Antibiotics Can Lead to Cancer

For many people around the world, antibiotics have saved lives and revolutionized health care. However, not all is as rosy as one would think in the world of antibiotics.

In Washington State, U.S., a study was done on the association between the use of antibiotics and the risk of breast cancer. Dr. Christine Velicer Ph.D., led the study, which included 2,266 women with primary, invasive breast cancer and 7,953 randomly selected females who did not have breast cancer. As these women were from a large nonprofit health plan, data on their antibiotic use was available.

The risk was smaller for women who took fewer antibiotics, but even women who had between one and 25 prescriptions, or had cumulatively used antibiotics for 1 to 500 days over an average period of 17 years, had an increased risk. They were about 150% more likely to be diagnosed with breast cancer than those women who didn't take any antibiotics.

A Canadian study looked at 3,099 people with breast cancer and compared them to 12,396 people who did not have breast cancer. It found that breast cancer rates were higher in people who had more antibiotic prescriptions during the 1 to 15 years before the study.

A 2008 study of 3,000,000 people divided the participants into groups that had taken no antibiotics for two years previous, those who had taken 2-5 prescriptions and those who had taken six or more prescriptions. Participants were tracked for six years afterwards.

Those who had taken 2-5 antibiotic prescriptions had a 27% increase in cancers compared to those who took none. Those who took six or more prescriptions had a 37% increase in cancers.

What is the connection between antibiotic use and breast cancer? One theory is that antibiotics interfere with the body's ability to properly break down and use cancer-fighting foods, due to the effect of antibiotics on the digestive system.

It's also possible that the use of antibiotics is simply a reflection of other immune system issues that are responsible for an increase in breast cancer. To date, most researchers would say that the findings required further study. However, a better understanding of how antibiotics work in your body may clear up some of the mystery.

While many people see antibiotics as the cure-all for every condition, you need to know that antibiotics kill the good, along with the bad. Your intestinal tract is a delicate balance of organisms, which need to function properly for you to have ideal health.

Wide-spectrum antibiotics, such as penicillin, go in like guerilla warfare and kill everything in sight. This can cause all sorts of problems such as vitamin deficiencies, loss of minerals, inflammation of the intestine, parasites, hormonal imbalances and even the development of food allergies.

Antibiotics also take out the immune system. The system we need so desperately to fight cancer, inflammation and infection actually gets suppressed while taking antibiotics. People who take antibiotics have more repeat infections than those who are not treated. Dr. Lawrence Wilson, MD, and nutritional consultant for 29 years says: "Antibiotics do not aid the immune system. They replace one of its functions. Antibiotics act by inhibiting certain enzymatic processes of bacteria, and by changing mineral balances. Normal cells, however, are also affected. This may be one reason why antibiotics weaken the immune response."

Antibiotics also contribute to the overgrowth of candida. Once an antibiotic starts messing around with that delicate balance in the intestines, candida takes over and creates problems.

One of the prime risk factors for chronic candida infection is repeated antibiotic use. As you learned in the chapter on candida, this can cause all sorts of problems, even cancer.

So are antibiotics bad? No, there may be times when an antibiotic would be the best medicine and could save your life. However, even doctors are now becoming alarmed at the over-use and the over-prescribing of antibiotics, which are causing problems such as the development of antibiotic-resistant super bugs. The sci-fi movies of the world being taken over by bacteria that no longer respond to antibiotics is actually far more realistic than people would like to believe.

Part of the problem is that antibiotics are prescribed for conditions that do not require an antibiotic. People assume anything and every-thing can be fixed with an antibiotic and can actually feel "not taken care of adequately" by the doctor if an antibiotic isn't given for every sniffle, cough or infection. You need to seriously look at antibiotics as having an intended purpose that is specific, not as a "fix-everything" pill to pop.

You also need to appreciate that everything from poultry, to beef, to farmed fish to dairy products, today, may be injected with antibiotics. Seventy percent of all antibiotics consumed in the U.S.—24 million pounds of antibiotics per year—goes into animals, and more than half of the antibiotics used are identical to those used in humans. While Europe has banned such use, it is still common practice in many countries, including the U.S.

Some of those antibiotics are making their way into the food system and into your body. This is why it is so important to carefully look at your diet, because you're being medicated just by eating a meal.

When you view your body as an amazingly intricate machine that is precisely tuned for optimum function, you respect the complexity of the systems in place to protect your health. Dr. Abelson, DC, RNC, reminds us that "there are benefits of letting our own immune system fight off infections. Most people have never realized that every time they fight off an infection, their immune system gets stronger. It is also important for us to realize that overuse of antibiotics can render the antibiotic ineffective in a true life threatening infection. In all cases, patients should always ask their physician for a swab test, and should always avoid broad-spectrum antibiotics. Finally, with any antibiotic treatment, make sure you replace the normal flora that the antibiotics have destroyed. Otherwise you remain susceptible to new infections and will set yourself up for everything from food allergies to hormonal imbalances." If you need to take antibiotics for any reason, then you will definitely want to take the Plexus Pro Bio5 as part of your health program to rebuild your intestinal flora.

Just as the finest timepieces are precisely tuned, your body is comprised of many delicate systems that are easily thrown off balance by antibiotics. Although antibiotics may be necessary at times, it should be your primary goal to repair and restore your immune system naturally. By doing so, antibiotics will be a rare event in your life, possibly never needed. That way your immune and digestive systems don't have to fight another enemy, taking them away from the critical daily battle of protecting you from cancer and maintaining optimum breast health.

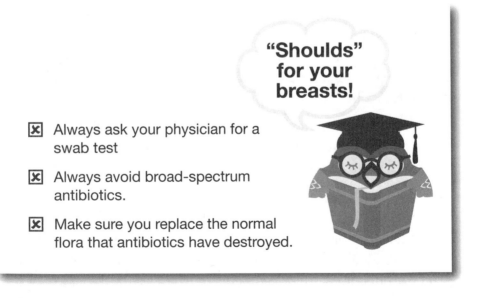

"Shoulds" for your breasts!

- ☒ Always ask your physician for a swab test

- ☒ Always avoid broad-spectrum antibiotics.

- ☒ Make sure you replace the normal flora that antibiotics have destroyed.

Secret #21:

The Scoop on Poop

Bowel movements are probably one of the least talked about subjects. Even doctors will usually just ask: Are your bowel movements regular? and leave it at that. If you're anything like me, you just say "yes," and hope they move on quickly.

Two of my dearest friends are colon queens. One has been a nutritionist for 29 years, the other a registered nurse for 30 years and a colon educator. They both love talking about poop. What it should look like, how it should smell (or not), how often it should happen and all the other stuff I definitely had filed in my "I don't really want to know about this" file.

However, over the years, it's been hard to duck their questions and concerns over my bowels, although I have really tried! What I have learned has been life changing, and I no longer squirm over this more delicate subject.

Bowel function is important. It's how your body gets rid of waste. Unfortunately, many people in developed countries simply don't have proper bowel function and have learned to live with it. However, a more accurate statement is that they are learning to die with it.

Brenda Eastwood, nutritionist, says proper bowel function should include:

- 2 -3 bowel movements per day (one per meal). You do not have to have a movement following each meal, but you must eliminate 2 to 3 times per day, which could all be in the morning or could all be in the evening.

- There should be no stress or straining.
- The total stool length per movement should measure from the crease of your wrist to the bend of your elbow. (This is when I am glad I have short arms.)
- The diameter should be the size of the circle you make by placing your pointer finger at the bend in your thumb.
- The stool should be light to medium brown in color, free of undigested food, non-odorous and mostly floating.

If you are saying, "holy moly," are you serious? then that is probably a big clue you have some work in this area. Honestly, most people do. I have eaten more fiber than just about anybody I know, having consumed a mostly vegetarian diet for 35 years, and I still had work to do in this arena. So don't feel bad if you are lacking in your bowel movements. Just know that you can never enjoy optimal health with an intestine full of you-know-what.

What does your poop have to do with breast health? Again, who would have thought they were connected, but they most definitely are.

Physicians Nicholas L. Petrakis and Eileen B. King of the University of California, have found that *women who have two or fewer bowel movements per week have four times the risk of breast disease* (benign or malignant) as women who have one or more bowel movements per day.

Dr. Petrakis reports, "We found that 5% of women having one bowel movement per day would have abnormal dysplastic cells, while 10% of women having fewer than one bowel movement a day would have this abnormality and 20% of women having two or fewer bowel movements per week would show these dysplastic changes in cell character of the breast fluid."

Why is there a correlation between your bowels and your breasts? One suggestion is: because estrogen is an established risk factor for breast cancer, the more bowel movements, the more estrogen excreted.

In another study of 28,586 postmenopausal women, ages 50-76 years, researchers observed a 46% decrease in breast cancer risk among women reporting very frequent (more than three bowel movements per day) than those reporting one bowel movement per day.

"The longer stool stays in the colon, the more one reabsorbs the metabolic products [such as estrogen] that have been excreted in the bile," says Dr. Patrick Donovan, who treats people with cancer in his naturopathic clinic. "We can see increased risk of breast cancer in women with a history of constipation."

With a very different twist on the subject, Melanie Ferreira, nutritionist looks beyond physical health: "The act of digestion and elimination can be seen as a metaphor for our ability to absorb what is useful from our experiences and eliminate what is unnecessary or harmful, or what holds us back. If you have a healthy bowel movement each day, you're letting go of the past and bringing in the new."

In line with previous chapters in this book, defecating can hold emotional memories. For example, if you were punished as a child for defecating in an inappropriate place (such as bed), or at an inconvenient time for a parent, then the unpleasant or painful memories can cause constipation. If shame or fear was associated with having a bowel movement as a child, this too can lead to less than ideal bowel movements as an adult. So you may need to look beyond physical concerns to resolve bowel issues.

However, something as simple as exercising your colon by jumping on a rebounder can have tremendous physical results. As you age, your colon can lose its elasticity and get out of shape. Obviously you can't take your colon out of your body and exercise with it to tone it, but rebounding has a positive effect on colons, as it helps to regain the elasticity needed for proper bowel function.

A colon cleanse can be a great way to get a whole new lease on bowel function, as it will clear the path, literally, for healthier, more frequent bowel movements. Look for something that is gentle, natural and easy. Drugs or harsh chemicals need to be avoided, as your intestines may appear to be tough, but there is a delicate balance that needs to be maintained.

As we have discussed throughout this report, there are many, many factors that create disease, not just one. So if you're constipated, the intention is not to immediately proclaim yourself a prime candidate for breast cancer, but rather to look at your bowel function as an area that you need to spend some time improving.

Remember Dr. Welch's advice, "Pursuing disease is not at all the same as pursuing health. In fact, they easily conflict. It can be quite difficult to promote wellness when you are actively looking for things to be wrong."

I give you the facts because sometimes we need that wake-up call to action as a great motivator to do something. Unfortunately, we are so inundated with information these days, we need to get that our lack of action can result in serious consequences. So stay focused on your ultimate health while you take positive action.

Your colon is an important part of your body's detoxification, cleansing and elimination process. Just like a garbage can—if it gets beyond full to overflowing, you have a real mess on your hands. Your body will have the same problem if your bowels aren't operating properly. They too will overflow and expel the excess toxins through your skin, stinkier perspiration, or darker, smellier urine.

By maintaining ideal bowel function, you also help to keep the normal healthy bacteria in your intestinal tract in balance. This crucial process makes sure that the detoxification process of getting rid of excess hormones is completed and prevents estrogen dominance, which can lead to an increased risk of breast cancer. You may need to start with more vegetables to increase your fiber intake. You may need more pure water so your body has what it needs to make stool. Perhaps being more cognizant of recognizing your body's natural urges to defecate and honoring the body's time schedule, rather than your daytimer's schedule, is all you need. Whatever it takes to start having 2-3 bowel movements a day is your goal for optimum health.

Can you clearly see that what goes on with your bowels very definitely has an effect on your breasts? Isn't it really amazing how wonderfully we are made with all the pieces working together to keep our breasts happy and healthy?

A Salute to Healthy Breasts!

Have you learned a few things about your breast health? I hope that you got at least one or two "AHA moments." I encourage you to use this book as a constant reference to regain and maintain breast health.

There's just one tiny little thing I haven't yet shared with you. It has been scientifically proven that a vitamin supplement that stays on the shelf does not improve health, as my nutritionist friend Brenda Eastwood reminds her audiences. So too, reading this book without putting any of the 21 secrets into action will do nothing for you either.

Small steps can add up to amazing results over time. So just start with one small implementation and add one little thing each week.

We can make a huge impact simply by starting to take action. The healing of this planet is only going to happen with every one of us doing our part.

Breasts symbolize everything feminine, sacred and nurturing in the world. I believe that by committing to total breast health for every woman, man and child, everything will change, because it would have to.

Physically, we would feel thousands of times better, but our emotional and mental health would also dramatically improve. Our spiritual lives would soar and our financial freedom would be unparalleled. Is that all possible through optimum breast health for every woman, man and child? I believe yes. But we will need to take action.

The time has come to raise our voices and bring about urgently needed changes to protect ourselves (and our children) from the toxic, chemical-laden, hormone-ridden society we have come to accept as normal.

In 1978, Israel experienced a public outcry and was threatened with legal action resulting in the banning of many toxic chemicals such as DDT and PCB's that were directly linked in a 1976 study with breast cancer in women. Once Israel banned these chemicals, they began noting a significant decrease in the level of toxic chemicals found in human breast milk. Over the next 10 years, the rate of breast cancer deaths dropped sharply, with a 30 percent drop in mortality for women under 44 years old, and an 8 percent overall decline.

Stories like this excite me, as well as confirm for me that we can do something. Already so many amazing women and men are doing incredible things to make this world a better, safer place for our breasts and our children's breasts.

Know that you, too, can make a difference. First of all, start by applying one thing you learned in *Breast Health Exposed* to better your breast health. Whether it be eliminating a toxic substance from your daily regime, drinking more water, throwing out the soda pop or taking off your bra when you get home from work, you can have happier, healthier breasts starting today.

Secondly, you can give this book to other women and men that you know and care about. Think of five people you know and love today that you want to have this vital information. Gift it for birthdays and Christmas to women you love.

Thirdly, let people know about www.breasthealthrevolution.com, a website where you can take breast health back into your own hands and receive the education so desperately needed.

If someone gifted or loaned you this book, let them know how much you appreciated the vital information. Share your "AHA moments" with them. Tell them you are glad they cared enough to take action.

Together we can make a massive difference. Together we can have healthy breasts for every man, woman and child!

To Your Ultimate Breast Health,

Jan

Coming Spring 2011

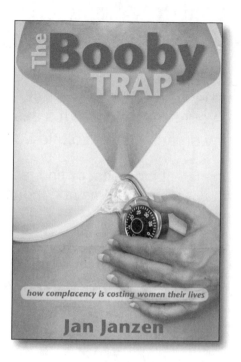

Why is it that the 21 secrets to achieving
breast health are not taught in schools,
promoted by major charities and
practiced in our medical system?

Find out the shocking truth about why
breast cancer has not been cured in
*The Booby Trap: How Complacency
is Costing Women Their Lives*

Want to Know More About Breast Health?

Stay up-to-date, informed and proactive when it comes to your breast health! It's easy to do at www.breasthealthrevolution.com

Read the latest blog post or find resources that will save you time and money!

Want to make a difference in the world of breast health?

Love Your Breasts Today!

Under 'Taking Action' you will find various ways you can contribute to happy, healthy breasts for every woman. The 22 campaign is just one way you can be part of the movement in a positive and easy way.

If you want to learn more about Plexus breast health products visit www.plexuspink.com